Tuberculosis in India

Status and Socioeconomic Aspects

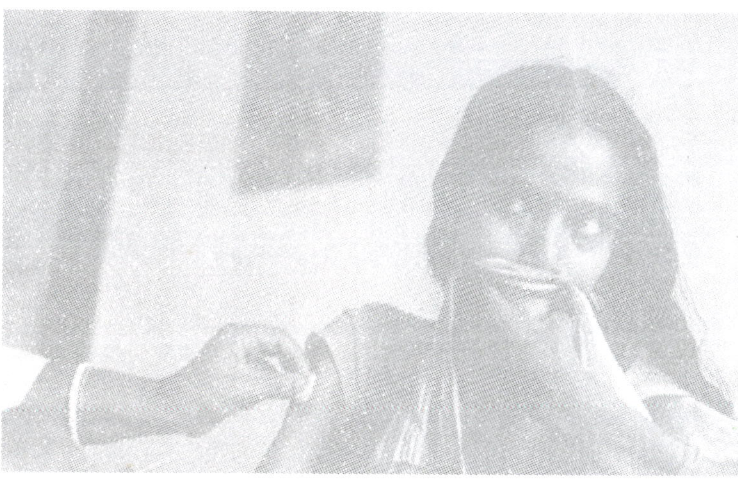

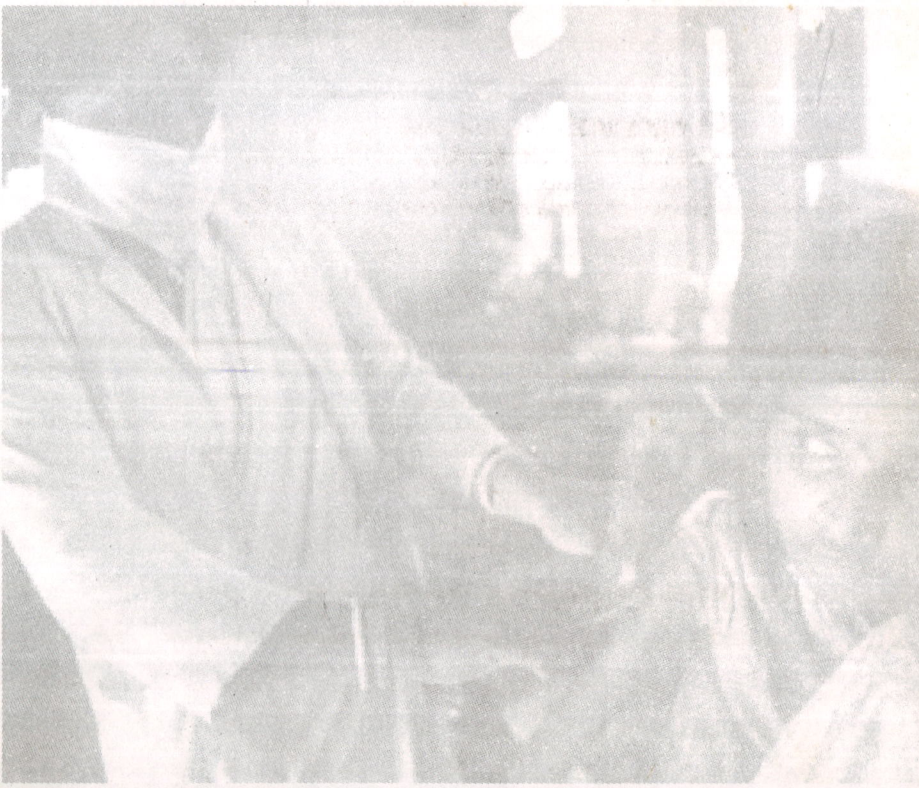

Tuberculosis in India

Status and Socioeconomic Aspects

ML Srivastava PhD
Ex-Professor of Demography and
Chief Technical Advisor
United Nations Organization

PC Bansil PhD
Director
Techno-Economic Research Institute
New Delhi

SP Agarwal MS, MCh, DSc (Hon)
Secretary General, Indian Red Cross Society and
Ex-Director General Health Services
Government of India, New Delhi

CBS

CBS Publishers & Distributors Pvt Ltd
New Delhi • Bengaluru • Pune • Kochi • Chennai

Tuberculosis in India
Status and Socioeconomic Aspects

ISBN: 978-81-239-2026-9

First Edition: 2012

Published by Satish Kumar Jain and produced by Vinod K. Jain for
CBS Publishers & Distributors Pvt Ltd
4819/XI Prahlad Street, 24 Ansari Road, Daryaganj
New Delhi 110 002, India.
Ph: 23289259, 23266861, 23266867
Fax: 011-23243014
Website: www.cbspd.com
e-mail: delhi@cbspd.com
cbspubs@airtelmail.in.

Branches

- Bengaluru: Seema House 2975, 17th Cross, K.R. Road, Banasankari 2nd Stage, Bengaluru 560 070, Karnataka
  Ph: +91-80-26771678/79 Fax: +91-80-26771680 e-mail: bangalore@cbspd.com
- Pune: Bhuruk Prestige, Sr. No. 52/12/2+1+3/2 Narhe, Haveli (Near Katraj-Dehu Road Bypass), Pune 411 051, Maharashtra
  Ph: 020-64704058, 64704059, 32392277 Fax: +91-020-24300160 e-mail: pune@cbspd.com
- Kochi: 36/14 Kalluvilakam, Lissie Hospital Road, Kochi 682 018, Kerala
  Ph: +91-484-4059061-65 Fax: +91-484-4059065 e-mail: cochin@cbspd.com
- Chennai: 20, West Park Road, Shenoy Nagar, Chennai 600 030, Tamil Nadu
  Ph: +91-44-26260666, 26208620 Fax: +91-44-45530020 email: chennai@cbspd.com

Printed at India Binding House, Noida (UP)

Preface

The infectious nature and wide prevalence of tuberculosis, the disease which has many peculiarities of its own in the shape of misinformation, nonpragmatic management and social stigmas, has remained one of the most serious concerns of humanity ever since the civilization began. Individuals, communities, scientists, planners and administrators have been busy all the time in battling against tuberculosis and striving to get control over it. Despite the availability of drugs (for over 50 years) to completely cure the disease, we have not been able to eradicate the disease from the world. The Central TB Division of the Directorate General of Health Services, Ministry of Health and Family Welfare, Government of India, sponsored a field survey based study with the objective to assess the socioeconomic implications of tuberculosis on patients and their families living in the state of Delhi. The study, carried out during the period 2005–06 at the Techno-Economic Research Institute, was designed to provide a baseline data for effective and efficient planning and implementation of India's current national tuberculosis control programme.

Although the study was intended to cover the limited objective as above, the Institute collected a lot of additional information beyond the six questionnaires used in the field work. After completing the report on the research assignment, authors felt the need to not only make full use of the material collected but also to make a comprehensive treatise on tuberculosis. The present book is an attempt in this direction. It caters to a wider readership ranging from a common man interested in knowing about various aspects of the disease in a nontechnical manner to the serious scholars, community leaders, planners, administrators, service providers and others interested in quantitative and qualitative assessment of incidence, prevalence, management, control and implications of the disease on our individual and collective lives.

The book is divided into two parts, respectively containing four and seven chapters. Chapter 1 gives a detailed picture of the disease in a largely nontechnical but informative manner from the perspective of a common reader. The topics include nature and types of tuberculosis, method of invasion and attack, progression, prevention, detection, diagnosis and treatment. It also includes topics relevant to know its connection with HIV/AIDS and mutation to drug resistant form of the disease and its treatment. Since the disease appears to be a part of our common history, it may be interesting to know the historical developments related to identification, nomenclature, prevention and control through which the disease had to pass and the efforts that were made to control and eradicate it. Chapter 2 that covers this aspect traces the historical developments at the international level, separated into ancient, medieval and modern periods. The concluding section of the chapter presents the historical developments related to the disease in India. The data on the incidence and the prevalence is essential to provide a quantitative picture of the burden of the disease that has posed such difficulties through the ages. This aspect is taken up in Chapter 3. It summarizes the extent of the disease in India as compared to selected countries, the regions and in the world at large. Chapter 4 deals with the current status of management and control of the disease at the international and national levels. It covers the description of the status of various strategies for controlling and eradicating the disease in the country.

The success of any programme to prevent, control and treat tuberculosis largely depends upon the perception of the problem by patients, their families and the community they live in and the pragmatic action taken by authorities to rectify them. This required an adequate data base which could help discern the implications of the disease on a holistic basis involving economic and social factors and to help design a programme for addressing them efficiently and effectively. Part II of the book highlights the economic and social-psychological implications of the disease along with quality of service provisions and status of client's satisfaction. The background to and justification for case study presented here are given in Chapter 5 whereas the status of tuberculosis in Delhi as revealed by official data and household surveys is given in Chapter 6. Various aspects of methodology and profile of sample population are given in Chapter 7.

The study covers topics, such as the socioeconomic profile, treatment-seeking behaviour, social costs, economic costs, financial burden of the disease, profile of service providers, and level of patients' satisfaction. The study was limited to patients who were attending the government facilities. Treatment-seeking behaviour is the most important element of a programme to control a disease like tuberculosis which is infectious and may perpetuate even after cure. The treatment-seeking behaviour, however, depends upon a number of characteristics of individual users. These aspects are covered in Chapter 8. Tuberculosis is associated with several stigmas generally linked to its debilitating effects which, in turn, brings heavy economic burden, among others. The worst affected is the family. The present study examined the impact of the disease on the employment, working hours, job change, income, duration of treatment, expenditure related to disease, financing of treatment, and financial burden of illness. These aspects are given in Chapter 9. Tuberculosis usually inflicts quite heavy toll on social life and psychological conditions of the patient. The patient experiences some sort of mental torture and social isolation. Understanding of the extent of such experiences is expected to help design and implement programmes to counter them and facilitate the participation of patients and communities in the control and eventual eradication of the disease. The case study examined all these issues ranging from discrimination at various levels to treatment by family and other members of the community. Chapter 10 covers the findings.

The success of tuberculosis control programme largely depends upon the productive blend of available services and satisfaction of service users. This aspect was analysed with reference to location, infrastructure, quality and behaviour of service providers on the one hand and profile and satisfaction level of service users on the other. Chapter 11 summarizes the findings in respect of selected parameters.

ML Srivastava
PC Bansil
SP Agarwal

Acknowledgements

The Institute is grateful to the Central TB Division of the Directorate General of Health Services, Ministry of Health and Family Welfare, Government of India, for giving us an opportunity to undertake a thorough field study on this important subject. Dr LC Chauhan, the then Deputy Director (TB), deserves special thanks. He was available for fruitful discussions as and when required during the course of the study, despite his heavy office work. We had really very fruitful input from a high level technical committee during the course of the study. Our sincere thanks to Dr Padam Singh, Ex-Additional DG, Indian Council of Medical Research (Chairman); Dr SK Sharma, Professor and Head, Department of Medicine, All India Institute of Medical Sciences (Member); Dr VK Vijayan, Director, Patel Chest Institute, Delhi University (Member); Dr PP Mandal, CMO, Central TB Division, MOHFW, New Delhi (Member); and Dr Sai Kumar, WHO Consultant; for their contributions.

Constant guidance and consultation on all technical issues was provided by two highly qualified experts Dr Ashini Sirivastava (Public Health) and Dr Madhu Kanodia (TB specialist) who deserve our profound thanks.

Mohd. Assad Siddiqui and his team carried out the field work with utmost dedication and diligence. Without their contribution the study would not have succeeded to the extent it did. The field team deserves our grateful thanks.

The guidance and help received from Institute faculty members Mr BK Taimini (Ex-Food Secretary, GoI), Dr PN Radha Krishnan, Dr Padam Singh, Dr SR Mohnot and Prof SK Gupta is gratefully acknowledged. Their precious contributions helped in improving the quality of the study. The contribution of the Institute's team comprising Mr KR Dasgupta, Dr SS Sirohi and Mr CP Sharma is highly appreciated and acknowledged. Last, but certainly not the least, the total responsibility of providing office support fell on our two diligent staff members, Mrs Ajitha Gangatharan and Mrs Vasantha R Pillai, who cheerfully helped in the printing/reprinting of various draft reports from time to time.

This study is the revised, updated and expanded version of the original report which was hardly one-fifth the present size. The report is based on several published/unpublished sources. Although every effort has been made to acknowledge the source wherever possible, yet it could have been left out unintentionally at a few places. The views expressed and conclusions arrived at are, however, the total responsibility of the authors alone.

ML Srivastava
PC Bansil
SP Agarwal

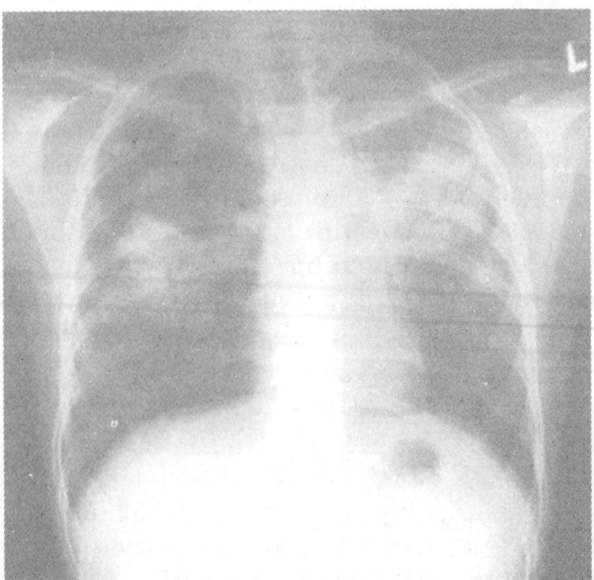

Contents

Part II SOCIOECONOMIC ASPECTS: A CASE STUDY OF DELHI

Part I

Status

1

The Disease

1.1 INTRODUCTION

Origin of Tuberculosis

Tuberculosis has a lineage that can be traced to the earliest history of mankind. Based on a number of archeological researches, the occurrence of disease has been noted in several countries at various times. Tuberculosis was prevalent in the animal kingdom long before it attacked mankind. The transition probably took the route from animals to mankind through milk ingestion after the domestication of animals. However, after 1000 BC there are evidences for widespread occurrence of pulmonary tuberculosis. The prevalence of the disease has been noted in several population groups across all the continents.

A recent study entitled "Predominance of Ancestral Lineages of *Mycobacterium Tuberculosis* in India" conducted jointly by a team of Indian and French scientists has shown that the ancestral strains of the TB bacterium was widespread in India. This finding indicated the possibility that India might be the ancient reservoir for TB, from which more recent strains evolved and spread to other countries.

The study considered 91 isolates from 12 different regions spread across the country. After analyzing the samples by genotyping with several tests, highly congruent groupings were found. Using four independent sets of markers, the study identified three lineages which corresponded to the ancestral strain. These were: an East African Indian, Delhi and the more modern and virulent Beijing geno-groups. To study the diversity, strains from patients in India between 1997 and 2002 were considered. The researchers observed an excellent congruence between the four independent sets of markers and concluded on the nature of different prevalent lineages.

Most of the Indians were found to be suffering from the treatable and less harmful ancestral TB virus. This conclusion implies that India is the origin for the disease. The virulent modern strain, Beijing strain, is present in very few numbers. The study has been extended to cover the impact of migration of Indians suffering from TB to other countries[1]. More details about the history are given at another place in this book.

Disease as understood Today

Tuberculosis (TB) is an airborne infectious disease caused by the *Mycobacterium tuberculosis*. An acute or chronic infectious disease of humans and various animals, it is caused by bacteria of the genus Mycobacterium, often called tubercle bacilli. The bacillus infects the lungs by inhalation of infected droplets formed during coughing of an individual with the active form of the disease. In the vast majority of the cases the infection is localized and without any symptom, but it may progress to cause chronic pulmonary tuberculosis. Human infection with *M. tuberculosis* was one of the leading cause of death until anti-tuberculosis drugs were introduced in the 1940s.

It mostly affects the lungs (pulmonary TB) but can also affect other parts of the body such as heart, kidney, central nervous system (meningitis), lymphatic system, circulatory system, genitourinary system, reproductive system, bones, skin and joints.

Tuberculosis is one of the most deadly and common major infectious diseases today, infecting about two billion people or one-third of the world's population. Nine million new cases of disease, resulting in two million deaths, occur annually, mostly in developing countries.

The disease in man is caused either by the human or by the bovine type of tubercle bacillus. Bacilli of the human type are

---

[1]Times of India, January 15, 2007.

spread by the cough spray and expectoration of sufferers from pulmonary tuberculosis, and reach the lung via the air passages. Bacilli of bovine type are found in the milk of cows with udder tuberculosis, and enter the human body through the alimentary tract. Bacilli of either type may be carried to other parts of the body.

There is a difference between being infected with the TB bacterium and having active tuberculosis disease. The predominant TB bacterium is *Mycobacterium tuberculosis* (*M. tuberculosis*). Most people infected with *M. tuberculosis* never develop active TB. However, in people with weakened immune systems, especially those with HIV (human immunodeficiency virus), TB organisms can overcome the body's defenses, multiply, and cause an active disease.

Tuberculosis and Animals

Although our primary interest here lies in the description of the human strain of tuberculosis, it may be worthwhile to note that the disease is also found in the animal kingdom where most of the species appear to be susceptible to the disease linked mainly to three strains of *Mycobacterium tuberculosis.*

The first and the most important one of these strains, *the bovine strain*, causes most cases of generalized tuberculosis in cattle, pigs, horses and cats, many cases in dogs, and rare cases in sheep and goats. The other two strains, *the human type* and *the avian type*, have generally low severity and virulence for domestic animals and primates. However, sometimes it can produce progressive tuberculosis in cattle, pigs and horses. There is another strain that affects reptiles and fish but does not appear to infect the mammals under natural conditions.

Tuberculosis is a matter of serious concern in cattle particularly dairy cattle. The disease spreads easily among such animals and becomes progressive where dairy cattle are kept under confined and demanding conditions. The mortality of such animals becomes a hazard to human health directly through contact or indirectly through consumption of un-pasteurized milk.

Tuberculosis in horses has never been common. It is rarer in sheep and goats. Progressive tuberculosis in pigs usually due to bovine strain may be acquired from cattle. It can sometimes be caused by avian strain but resulting lesions are generally localized. Tuberculosis in poultry is not common as it used to be earlier and it is found mostly in individual birds kept under overcrowded and unhygienic conditions. The disease has also been seen among the wild birds, namely, pheasants, wood pigeons, sparrows, sea gulls, starlings etc. Dogs are susceptible to infection with human and bovine strains. This may happen through human contact or from milk. In the case of cats there is resistance to infection from the human strain and most cases are due to bovine strain, probably from milk.

Tuberculosis can be carried by many mammals. Domesticated species, such as cats and dogs, are generally free of tuberculosis, but wild animals may be carriers. As a result, many places have regulations restricting the ownership of novelty pets, possibly including such partially domesticated species such as pet skunks; for example, the American state of California forbids the ownership of pet gerbils. The strictness of such restrictions generally depends on the public health policies adopted for fighting tuberculosis. Developed countries have organized programmes to eradicate bovine tuberculosis. The efforts have largely been concentrated in cattle population.

TB Knows Colours[2]

People with dark skins are more susceptible to tuberculosis. A recent study reported in online version of Science on February 23, 2006, showed that low level of vitamin D in people with dark skin is likely to make this happen. Scientists studied the response of human immune cells to tuberculosis bacteria and found that the germs stimulate a set of receptors present on these cells. This triggers a set of reactions—the cells produce an enzyme that activates vitamin D to manufacture a protein that can kill the germs.

Dark skin people have high levels of melanin—the pigment that provides colour to skin. This melanin reduces the skin's

[2]Science, online version, February 23, 2006.

ability to produce vitamin D. When exposed to the bacteria, cells cultured in blood samples taken from dark-skinned people produced about one-third of the microbe-killing protein produced by fair-skinned people. Supplementing the samples from dark-skinned people with a vitamin D precursor boosted the production of the protective protein.

Active Tuberculosis

A person has active tuberculosis when the bacteria in one's body are actively multiplying. She/he has one or more symptoms of the disease and can spread it to other people. One in ten people that are infected with *M. tuberculosis* may develop active TB at some time in their lives. The risk of developing active disease is greatest in the first year after infection, but active disease often does not occur until many years later. Early symptoms of active TB can include weight loss, fever, night sweats, and loss of appetite, or they may be vague and go unnoticed by the affected individuals. One in three patients with TB will die within weeks to months if the disease is not treated. For the rest, their disease either goes into remission (halts) or becomes chronic and more debilitating with cough, chest pain, and bloody sputum. Symptoms of TB involving areas other than the lungs vary, depending upon the organ affected.

Latent Tuberculosis

Latent tuberculosis is when a person is infected with *Mycobacterium tuberculosis*, but does not develop active disease. The body's immune system is able to wall off the bacteria and contain it under a protective coat of scar tissue. Patients with latent tuberculosis are not infectious, and do not have any symptoms of the disease. The main risk is that approximately a quarter of these patients will go on to develop active tuberculosis at a later stage of their life. The identification and treatment of people with latent TB is an important part of controlling this disease.

1.2 TYPES OF TUBERCULOSIS

Tuberculosis may broadly be classified into two groups- pulmonary and non-pulmonary.

Pulmonary tuberculosis, as the name signifies, most commonly affects the lungs (75% or more). Symptoms of the disease include a productive, prolonged cough of more than three weeks duration, chest pain, and hemoptysis (coughing up blood). Systemic symptoms include fever, chills, night sweats, appetite loss, weight loss, and easy fatigability. Additional symptoms include occasional massive hemorrhages when lung tissue is destroyed by the disease and collection of fluid in the pleural cavity. The use of the term consumption to designate this disease arose because sufferers appeared as if they were "consumed" from within by the disease. People from Asian and African descent may have more often lymph node TB than Caucasians. Individuals may experience these symptoms differently. These should be taken as cautionary and not as definitive.

Pulmonary tuberculosis develops from minute lesions caused by primary lung tuberculosis infection when bacteria enter the lungs through air passages and multiply causing a local lung infection. The local lymph node around the lungs may also get involved and become enlarged. Notably, the hilar lymph nodes (the lymph nodes adjacent to the heart) at the base of the lungs often become enlarged. In case these lesions do not heal, an area of progressive disease, detectable by X-ray examination, may develop around them. This sequence of events that occurs after the first exposure to bacteria is termed 'primary tuberculosis'. In most cases the immune system can resist the attack and make a protective wall around the area of infection. This scar tissue later calcifies and can be seen as stony deposit on X-ray examination. In more unfavourable instances, primary tuberculosis may spread locally and sometimes actually in the lungs from invasion of the bronchial tree by the bacilli. It may be disseminated by the blood stream to other parts of the body. Pleurisy may occur as an early sequel to primary infection, particularly among young people. Progressive pulmonary tuberculosis in adolescents and adults may, as in young children, start by local spread from a recent lesion. This is probably becoming more common as primary infection takes place later in life. Most usually, however, the disease is 'post-primary' starting in the upper part of one or both lungs as a fresh re-infection originating from outside or from within.

There is wide variation in the forms of pulmonary tuberculosis in different racial groups. For example, in parts of Africa it tends to be acute, extensive and often bilateral whereas in southern India, it tends to acquire chronic forms as in Europe. However, the lesions in the former group are usually more advanced than in the latter. There is a possibility for these differences to be connected to the local evolution of the disease which may be a temporary trend.

Non-pulmonary Tuberculosis

Extra-pulmonary sites include the pleura, central nervous system (meningitis), lymphatic system (scrofula of the neck), genitourinary system, and bones and joints (Pott's disease of the spine). An especially serious form is "disseminated", or "miliary" TB, so named because the lung lesions so-formed resemble millet seeds on X-ray. These are more common in immunosuppressed persons and in young children. Pulmonary TB may co-exist with extra-pulmonary TB.

In developed countries where tuberculosis in man is declining and tuberculosis infection from milk has been suppressed, non-pulmonary tuberculosis involving bones, joints and lymph nodes (e.g. glands in the neck) is becoming rare. In developing countries, on the other hand, the disease, though overshadowed by the much larger figures for pulmonary disease, is still a considerable problem. Non-pulmonary tuberculosis is much less infectious than pulmonary one, since bacilli in the former case are not usually coughed out.

Genital TB[3]

Tuberculosis of reproductive parts in which fallopian tubes get affected makes many Indian women infertile. The disease remains undetected due to lack of awareness and the absence of well-defined symptoms. Tubal factor infertility forms a major

[3]Savita Verma, Mail Today, April 14.

subset of patients who require assisted reproduction. The study carried out by the All India Institute of Medical Sciences found that genital TB was responsible for close to 50% of the cases of infertility.

Genital TB was thought to be on the decline but prevalence studies showed it was still a major contributor of tubal factor infertility. This form of TB continues to be ignored in the TB control programmes. Early diagnosis is difficult because of lack of specific symptoms. By the time the patients reach the doctor the fallopian tube are already blocked and infertility becomes irreversible. Information Education Communication components of tuberculosis control programmes should include advisory services where families with history of TB should get tested for the disease. The disease occurs when primary tuberculosis infection remains neglected and untreated, which leads to spread of the disease to reproductive system. It is a disease of developing countries. In developed countries genital tuberculosis has been found only in small number of infertile patients. In US one per cent of infertile patients have genital tuberculosis while in Italy, 0.8% of the infertile patients have the disease.

1.3 TRANSMISSION (METHOD OF INVASION)

Transmission of infectious TB usually occurs by an aerosol route. It can only occur from people with active TB disease (not latent TB infection). The disease can also spread through the gastrointestinal tract. People with active TB disease of the lungs while coughing, sneezing, speaking, or spitting expel droplet nuclei. Each droplet contains one to three bacilli which can remain suspended in the air for several hours. This process can also take place in the case of animals with active TB. Infection occurs if inhalation results in the organism(s) reaching the alveolus of the lungs. However, most of those infected (90%) have asymptomatic latent TB infection (LTBI). There is a 10% lifetime chance that LTBI will progress to active TB disease which, if left untreated, will kill more than 50% of its victims. TB is one of the top three infectious killing diseases in the world: AIDS and malaria are the other two. In specific subpopulation groups, however, such as infants, elderly, and persons with immunodeficiency status, the proportion who develop clinical TB is much higher. Further, some specific groups of people are at higher risk of developing the disease. Close contacts (people with prolonged, frequent, or intense contact) are at highest risk of becoming infected (typically a 22% infection rate).

The neglect of TB control programmes, HIV/AIDS, and immigration has caused a resurgence of tuberculosis. Multiple drug resistant strains of TB (MDR-TB) are emerging. The World Health Organization declared TB a global health emergency in 1993, and the *Stop TB Partnership* proposed a Global Plan to Stop Tuberculosis. By and large people of all ages, races, income levels, and both genders are likely to get TB infection. However, those at higher risk include the following:

- People who live or work with others who have TB.
- Medically underserved populations.
- Homeless people.
- People migrating from countries/areas where TB is prevalent.
- People in group settings, such as nursing homes.
- People from high-risk racial or ethnic minority population groups.
- Alcohol and intravenous drug users.
- People with impaired immune systems (HIV/AIDS).
- People who are poor and live in crowded settlements.
- The elderly.
- Children exposed to adults in high-risk categories.
- Healthcare workers who come in contact with high-risk populations.
- Drinking un-pasteurized milk.

It usually takes lengthy contact with someone with active TB before a person can become infected. On average, people have a 50 percent chance of becoming infected with *M. tuberculosis* if they spend eight hours a day for six months or 24 hours a day for two months working or living with someone with active TB. However, people with TB who have been treated with appropriate drugs for at least two weeks are no longer contagious and do not spread the germ to others. This high chance of transmission of TB is likely to be minimized or prevented by providing adequate ventilation in the living place.

A person with untreated, active tuberculosis can infect an estimated 15–20 other people per year. The probability of transmission depends upon infectiousness of the person with TB (quantity expelled), environment of exposure, duration of exposure, and virulence of the organism. The chain of transmission can be controlled by isolating patients with active disease, starting effective anti-tuberculous therapy, providing adequate ventilation in the living space and close monitoring of persons on anti-tubercular therapy. *M. bovis* transmission from cattle to humans has occurred through drinking contaminated milk. Nearly all cattle infected with *M. bovis* develop active disease and can transmit the organism to other animals and humans.

1.4 PATHOGENESIS (METHOD OF ATTACK)

The pathogenesis of tubercular infection and disease begins in most cases with the inhalation of the tubercle bacilli. TB infection begins when bacilli reach the pulmonary alveoli. The mycobacteria replicate exponentially. Subsequently bacteria are picked up by dendritic cells, which can transport the bacilli to local lymph nodes, and then through the bloodstream to the more distant tissues and organs where TB disease could potentially develop: lung apices, peripheral lymph nodes, kidneys, brain, and bone. Most of the disseminated lesions heal; although reactivation can cause miliary or meningeal tuberculosis. The primary site of infection in the lungs is called the Ghon focus.

A recent study has shown that TB Bacteria hijack 'fat route' for spreading[4]. Researchers at Cornell University have found that the TB-causing bacteria hijack the fat metabolism or take a 'fat route' for triggering latent tuberculosis infection to progress into active disease. The research shows that *Mycobacterium tuberculosis* (MTB) is able to stimulate the immune cells the bacterium infects to accumulate fat droplets, turning them into 'foamy' cells. Following initial infection the infected immune cells in the body clump together in the lungs in a cellular mass that is surrounded by a fibrous cuff. This

[4]TB Bacteria hijack 'fat route' for spreading, The Times of India, March 30, 2010.

structure, called a tubercle, physically protects the bacteria from being destroyed by the immune system and allows them to persist inside the host for years during a latent period when the host shows no symptoms of the disease.

The respiratory infection is reactivated only in a small percentage of individuals in whom it progressively destroys lung tissue. Very little is known about the exact causes of reactivation and the relative roles of the host and the pathogen. This finding could provide a major breakthrough for developing an effective treatment for tuberculosis.

Individuals who develop active disease either fail to contain the primary infection or develop reactivation as a result of relative or absolute immune suppression at a point remote from primary infection. This is most likely to occur in immuno competent adults within the first three years after exposure. Factors related to progression of disease reflect a weakened immune status and include inter-current disease or steroid-dependent disease or collagen vascular disease, poor nutritional status particularly related to alcohol and drug abuse, smoking, the extremes of age, and HIV infection.

Tuberculosis is classed as one of the granulomatous inflammatory conditions. The affected cells aggregate to form a granuloma which prevents dissemination of the mycobacteria and provides a local environment for communication of cells of the immune system. Bacteria are not eliminated with the granuloma. They become dormant and lead to a latent infection which can be diagnosed only by tuberculin skin test.

If TB bacteria gain entry to the blood stream from an area of tissue damage they spread through the body and set up many foci of infection, each appearing as tiny white tubercles in the tissues. This is called miliary tuberculosis and has a high case fatality. In many patients the infection waxes and wanes. Tissue destruction and necrosis are balanced by healing and fibrosis. Affected tissue is replaced by scarring and cavities filled with cheese-like white necrotic material. During active stage, some of the cavities are in continuity with the air passages bronchi and the material contained may be coughed up. It contains living bacteria and can pass on infection. Treatment with appropriate antibiotics kills bacteria and allows healing to take place. Affected areas are eventually replaced by scar tissue.

1.5 PROGRESSION

The TB bacterium is spread through the air; however, repeated exposure to the germs is usually necessary before a person will become infected. It is not likely to be transmitted through personal items, such as clothing, bedding, or other items that a person with TB has touched. Adequate ventilation is the most important measure to prevent the transmission of TB.

The progression of the disease goes through four important stages in sequence as follows:

- **Exposure:** This occurs when a person has been in contact, or exposed to, another person who is thought to have or does have TB. The probability of getting infection is dependent on the number of incident infectious cases in the community; the duration of their infectiousness; and the number and nature of interactions between the case and the contact per unit time of infectiousness, etc. Such a person will have a *negative skin test*, a normal chest X-ray, and no signs or symptoms of the disease.
- **TB infection:** This occurs when a person has the TB bacteria in his/her body, but does not have symptoms of the disease. This person would have a *positive skin test*, but a normal chest X-ray.
- **TB disease:** This describes the person that has signs and symptoms of an active infection. The person would have a positive skin test and a positive chest X-ray.
- **Death:** The disease when untreated advances to an early death of the infected person. Sometimes even after treatment death may occur but the chance of survival in the case of treatment is far greater than if not treated.

In those people in whom TB bacilli overcome the immune system defenses and begin to multiply, there is progression from TB infection to TB disease. This may occur soon after infection (primary TB disease 1 to 5%) or many years after infection (post primary TB, secondary TB, reactivation TB disease of dormant bacilli 5 to 9%). The risk of reactivation increases when immune system is compromised, such as that caused by infection with HIV. In patients co-infected with *M. tuberculosis* and HIV, the risk of reactivation increases to 10% per year, while in immune competent individuals, the risk is between 5 and 10% in a lifetime.

Between two to eight weeks after being infected with *M. tuberculosis*, a person's immune system responds to the TB germ by walling off infected cells. From then on the body maintains a standoff with the infection, sometimes for years. Most people undergo complete healing of their initial infection, and the bacteria eventually die off. A positive TB skin test, and old scars on a chest X-ray, may provide the only evidence of the infection. If, however, the body's resistance is low because of aging, infections such as HIV, malnutrition, or other reasons, the bacteria may break out of hiding and cause active TB.

About five percent of infected persons will develop TB disease in the first two years, and another five percent will develop disease later in life. In all, about 10% of infected persons with normal immune systems will develop TB disease in their lifetime. Some medical conditions increase the risk of progression to TB disease. In HIV infected persons with TB infection, the risk increases to 10% each year instead of 10% over a lifetime. Other such conditions include drug injection (mainly because of the life style of IV Drug users), substance abuse, recent TB infection (within two years) or history of inadequately treated TB, chest X-ray suggestive of previous TB, diabetes mellitus, silicosis, prolonged corticosteroid therapy and other immunosuppressive therapy, head and neck cancers, blood diseases (leukemia and Hodgkin's disease), end-stage renal disease, intestinal bypass, chronic malabsorption syndromes, or low body weight (10% or more below the ideal). Some drugs, including rheumatoid arthritis drugs may raise the risk of causing a latent infection to become active due to their interference with body's immune defense against TB.

1.6 PREVENTION OF TUBERCULOSIS

TB is largely a preventable disease. Prevention and control efforts may broadly be classified into three categories, namely, general, vaccines, and drug therapy. Also the efforts include the following priority strategies:

- Identification and treatment of all persons who have TB disease.
- Location and evaluation of persons who have been in contact with TB patients to determine whether they have TB infection or disease, and treat them appropriately.
- Testing of high-risk groups for TB infection to identify candidates for treatment of latent infection and to ensure the completion of treatment.
- In tropical areas where the incidence of atypical mycobacteria is high, exposure to nontuberculous mycobacteria gives some protection against TB.
- Use of special techniques such as ultraviolet light to sterilize the air, special filters, and special respirators and masks in hospitals and clinics.
- Isolation of TB patients in hospitals in special rooms with controlled ventilation and airflow.

General Measures

- Reduce the spread of infectious sputum and discourage spitting in public.
- Eradication of bovine tuberculosis.
- Efficiently planned case-finding, early diagnosis (by mass radiography of apparently healthy persons) and early treatment.
- Reduction in community overcrowding.
- Improvement in general standard of living and in dietary habits.

Specific Prevention by Vaccines

Successful BCG[5] vaccination is considered to give a substantial protection immunity that lasts for a few years. Introduced in 1924 in France, BCG was at first used for infants, especially those in tuberculous households. Later it was extended in many countries to any previously uninfected (tuberculin-negative) individual in a tuberculous environment at home or work who runs a more-than-average risk of developing the disease (e.g. nurses and medical students) and to the members of various groups in the ordinary population. Many countries use BCG vaccine as part of their TB control programs, especially for infants. The protective efficacy of BCG for preventing serious forms of TB (e.g. meningitis) in children is high (greater than 80%). However, the protective efficacy for preventing pulmonary TB in adolescents and adults is variable, from 0 to 80%. In a British Medical Research Council trial (1950 onwards) an 80% protection was shown in vaccinated urban 14–year–old school children to last at least six years and six months.

Since the World War II many millions have received the vaccine through the large-scale emergency projects in war-ravaged Europe and in many developing countries under the auspices of Scandinavian agencies, WHO and UNICEF, or through the routine schemes of the national authorities.

---

[5]Following the invention of Edward Jenner's smallpox vaccine, many doctors placed their hopes on developing a vaccine suitable to control tuberculosis. To this effect a less virulent strain of *M. tuberculosis* called *M. bovis* (the bovine strain of tuberculosis) was used. However, because of cattle to human transmission, *M. bovis* is equally contagious in humans. From 1908 to 1919, Calmette and Guérin in France serially passed M. bovis 230 times to result in a strain called acilli Calmette-Guérin, which is commonly called BCG. It is avirulent in cattle, horses, rabbits, and guinea pigs. First administered to humans in 1921, it is still applied today. However, due to various strains because the original stocks were not kept, it has been impossible to judge the efficiency of BCG. BCG is a live vaccine prepared from a strain of tubercle bacilli whose virulence is weakened so that it produces an infection without any harmful disease, the infection being indicated by a positive tuberculin test.

In the United Kingdom, children aged 10–14 were typically immunized during school until 2005. The effectiveness of BCG is much lower in areas where mycobacteria are less prevalent. In the USA, BCG vaccine is not routinely recommended except for selected persons who meet specific criteria.

In those parts of the world where the disease is common, the World Health Organization (WHO) recommends that infants receive a vaccine called BCG made from a live weakened bacterium related to *M. tuberculosis*. BCG vaccine prevents *M. tuberculosis* from spreading within the body, thus preventing TB from developing.

However, the vaccine has its drawbacks. It does not protect adults very well against TB. In addition, BCG interferes with the TB skin test, showing a positive skin test reaction in people who have received BCG vaccine. In countries where BCG vaccine is used, the ability of the skin test to identify persons that are infected with *M. tuberculosis* is limited. Because of these limitations, more effective vaccines are needed and BCG is not recommended for general use in the United States.

New TB Vaccine Offers Glimmer of Hope to HIV Positive People[6]

AUS National Institutes of Health sponsored research in Dar-es-Salaam, Republic of Tanzania, has developed a new Tuberculosis vaccine that can reduce the risk of HIV-infected people falling sick with TB. This was announced recently at the 39th Union World Conference on Lung Health in Paris by the Executive Director of the International Union against TB and Lung Diseases as the most exciting and promising development for people living with HIV (PLHIV) in recent times. When tested in a seven-year long study the vaccine was found to boost lymphocyte counts and protect against all forms of definite TB among 20 of the 1,000 who received it. The study did not point to any risk of getting TB infection from the vaccine itself as it was an inactivated form. The technology used to create the vaccine is low cost and that will help ensure its affordability in those countries where it will be needed most.

[6]The Hindu, New Delhi, October 24, 2008.

It's utility can be appreciated if we consider that one in five people with a severely weakened immune system can develop active TB within a year.

ATB vaccine that will afford permanent protection is badly needed. It is too early to know if the newly developed Myco-baterium vaccae vaccine, as it is designated, can do that. The follow-up with the study volunteers shows that the vaccine is affording a 40 per cent protection so far in these three to four years. There is a need to study its longer durability. The new vaccine is expected to have a profound impact on TB control among PLHIV in India as elsewhere. It is estimated that about 6,000 cases of TB can be averted among a population of 2 million PLHIV within three years if 50% of the patients received it. The current practice of preventing TB using the BCG vaccine given to children at birth protects them from acquiring serious TB it does not afford much protection to adults. Additionally, BCG being a live vaccine could theoretically cause TB in PLHIV. The only drug available for protecting such patients from TB is to give them a daily dose of a single anti-TB drug—Isoniazid. However, this practice is likely to increase the spread of Isoniazid resistant TB, but is still adopted as the lesser of the two evils. The new vaccine would overcome both these challenges. The potential of the new vaccine to prevent TB among HIV negative individuals in TB prevalent areas is open to exploration. Meantime, it may be two years before Myco-bacterium vaccae will become available.

The Mantoux Test

The Mantoux test (or Mantoux screening test, Tuberculin Sensitivity Test, Pirquet test, or PPD test for Purified Protein Derivative) is a diagnostic tool for tuberculosis and not the disease. This is so because all the infected persons may not develop active tuberculosis. With this test one can not be sure that one has tuberculosis. However, a negative result of the test suggests that one is free of the tuberculosis infection. In children sometimes it is useful. Efforts should be made to have definitive test.

The Mantoux test is used in the United States and is endorsed by the American Thoracic Society and Centers for Disease Control and Prevention (CDC).

Multiple puncture tests such as the Tine test are not recommended. The Mantoux test is one of the two major tuberculin skin tests for tuberculosis used in the world. The Heaf test is used in the United Kingdom and is endorsed by the British Thoracic Society.

BCG Vaccine and the Mantoux Test

Tuberculin skin testing is not contraindicated for BCG-vaccinated persons. Latent TB infection (LTBI) diagnosis and treatment for LTBI is considered for any BCG-vaccinated person whose skin test is 10 mm or greater, if any of these circumstances are present:

- Was in contact with another person with infectious TB.
- Was born or has lived in a high TB prevalence country.
- Is continually exposed to populations where TB prevalence is high.

Sponsored by the National Institute of Allergy and Infectious Diseases (NIAID), the first recombinant tuberculosis vaccine entered clinical trials in the United States in 2004. A 2005 study showed that a DNA TB vaccine given with conventional chemotherapy can accelerate the disappearance of bacteria in mice. Simultaneously it can also provide protection against re-infection. However, it may take four to five years for it to be available for use in humans.

Because of the limitations of current vaccines, researchers and policymakers are promoting new economic models of vaccine development including prizes, tax incentives and advance market commitments.

Chemoprophylaxis

This is a specific measure aimed at preventing tuberculous disease by giving anti-tuberculous drugs either to uninfected (tuberculin-negative) persons who are at a high risk of becoming infected (primary prophylaxis), or to persons already infected with the bacillus (giving positive reaction to the tuberculin skin test) but with no evidence of tuberculous disease (secondary prophylaxis). The drug generally used is isoniazid alone, on the presumption that the risk of drug resistance is negligible under these circumstances. As a measure for long-term mass administration to large numbers of healthy children, primary prophylaxis is probably unjustifiable, and even secondary prophylaxis is still considered controversial. There is a body of opinion in favour of the use of primary and secondary prophylaxis in children in overcrowded tuberculous households, possibly combined with BCG in those who are tuberculin-negative; secondary prophylaxis is also probably has a place for use in high-risk groups, e.g. in infected infants, and in adolescents showing strong reactivity to tuberculin though without detectable disease.

1.7 TUBERCULOSIS AND HIV INFECTION/AIDS

Sudden development of TB in any person may be one of the first indications that she or he is infected with HIV. This form of TB often occurs in areas outside the lungs, particularly when the patient is in the later stages of AIDS. It is noted that the disease frequently occurs early in the course of HIV infection, often months to years before other opportunistic infections such as *Pneumocystis carinii* pneumonia. In the United States, it is much more likely for persons infected with *M. tuberculosis* and HIV to develop active TB than it is for someone that is only infected with *M. tuberculosis*. However, TB disease can be prevented and cured, even in people with HIV infection. In the United States, a person co-infected with TB and HIV develops active disease at a rate of about 8 percent each year. By comparison, otherwise healthy individuals infected with *M. tuberculosis* have a 10 percent lifetime risk of developing active disease. People with HIV also are at greater risk of having a new infection progress directly to active disease.

TB is difficult to diagnose in those suffering from AIDS because such patients do not show all the symptoms of the disease. However, HIV infected patients frequently have conditions which show symptoms similar to those of TB, but may not react to the standard TB skin test because their immune system does not work properly. Although investigators have hypothesized that a two-stage TB skin test might be more reliable than a single-stage test in HIV-infected individuals, a recently completed NIAID study found this is not to be the case. X-rays, sputum tests, and physical examinations may also fail to provide evidence of infection with *M. tuberculosis* in HIV-infected individuals. Only a third of all TB smear tests in HIV-positive patients give an accurate positive result. As a consequence, doctors must often decide to begin anti-TB therapy in HIV-infected people suspected of having active disease while waiting for the results of cultures of sputum or other specimens.

Tuberculosis is the most common cause of deaths for AIDS patients. The World Health Organization (WHO) estimates that 10 million people worldwide are infected with the *M. tuberculosis* bacterium and HIV virus at the same time. The primary cause of death in these patients is from TB, not AIDS. In the United States, it is estimated that about 2 out of ten persons who have TB are also infected with HIV.

People with MDR-TB that are also infected with HIV appear to have a more rapid and deadly disease course than do those patients with MDR-TB who are otherwise healthy. If no medicines are available for these patients as many as eight out of ten may die, often within months of diagnosis.

Detection/Diagnosis

A complete medical evaluation for tuberculosis (TB) includes the following steps:

- Medical history and physical examination
- Tuberculin skin test
- A chest X-ray; and
- Microbiologic smears and cultures of sputum.

The *medical history* of the patient includes obtaining the history of duration of cough, sputum, blood in sputum, fever, night sweat, weight loss, chest pain, fatigue, and loss of appetite. Other parts of the medical history include prior TB exposure, infection or disease; past TB treatment; demographic risk factors for TB; and medical conditions that increase risk for TB disease such as HIV infection. Tuberculosis should be suspected when a persistent respiratory illness in an otherwise healthy individual does not respond to regular antibiotics.

In those instances where the advance of the disease remains undetected or unchecked, cough and expectoration increase, loss of weight and fatigue are progressive, breathing gets difficult, fever and night sweats may occur. Progressively other typical symptoms may appear which include sputum streaked with blood; sometimes massive hemorrhages occur as lung tissue is destroyed by the disease. Fluid may collect in the pleural cavity. Gradual deterioration occurs and, if the disease is untreated, death is common. Tuberculous laryngitis may complicate the picture, causing hoarseness.

Skin Test

The infection for *M. tuberculosis* in people who do not develop the disease can be detected by doctors with a TB skin test. In this test, a small amount of testing material (purified protein derived from the bacillus) is injected into the top layer of the skin. If a certain size red bump develops within 72 hours after the injection, the test may be positive indicating that the person being tested has a possible tuberculosis infection.

The bacilli can remain dormant for years before becoming active. Therefore a positive test does not necessarily mean that the person being tested has active disease. Most people with previous exposure to *M. tuberculosis* will test positive on the tuberculin test. Such results may also be noted among those who were exposed to bacteria that related to the TB germ.

TB skin tests are suggested for those:

- In high-risk categories.
- Who live or work in close contact with people who are at high-risk.
- Who have never had a TB skin test.

Recommendations for skin testing in children, according to the American Academy of Pediatrics are as follows:

Immediate Testing

- If the child is thought to have been exposed in the last 5 years.
- If the child has an X-ray that looks like TB.
- If the child has any symptoms of TB.
- If the child is coming from countries where TB is prevalent.

Yearly Skin Testing

- Children with HIV.
- Children that are in jail.

Testing Every 2 to 3 Years

- Children that are exposed to high-risk people.

Consider Testing in Children from Ages 4 to 6 and 11 to 16 if

- A child's parent has come from a high-risk country.
- A child has traveled to high-risk areas.
- Children who live in densely populated areas.

Chest X-Ray

Chest X-ray may show an old infection with scarring (fibrosis) or calcification in the lungs or may reveal active pulmonary TB with infiltrates or consolidation and/or cavities that are often seen in the upper lungs with or without involvement of surrounding lymph nodes. There may also be collection of fluid in the bases of the lungs (pleural effusion). However, lesions may appear anywhere in the lungs. In disseminated TB a pattern of many tiny nodules throughout the lung fields is common. In HIV and other immunosuppressed persons, any abnormality may indicate TB or the chest X-ray may even appear entirely normal. Abnormalities on chest radiographs may be suggestive of, but are never diagnostic of, TB. However, chest radiographs may be used to rule out the possibility of pulmonary TB in a person who has a positive reaction to the tuberculin skin test and no symptoms of disease.

Microbiologic smears and cultures: Additional tests may be needed to determine if a person has TB disease. In the case the affected organ is the lung, the diagnosis includes X-rays and sputum tests. If the test is carried out through mass radiography on presumed healthy groups it is more likely to detect the disease at an early stage. Sputum examination may show tubercle bacilli by direct smear (sputum spread on a slide) examination. Bacteria culture is a more reliable method of diagnosis. A small amount of sputum is allowed to grow in a special culture medium and within a few weeks it demonstrates the presence of TB bacteria that stain positive with a special dye. These bacteria are called acid fast bacteria (AFB). When the affected organ is other than the lung, culture material is taken out by biopsy carried out by a trained person.

Because *M. tuberculosis* grows very slowly, it can take four weeks to confirm the diagnosis. It takes an additional two to three weeks to determine antibiotic sensitivity of the bacteria.

Polymerase chain reaction: Newer tests like polymerase chain reaction that test the genetic material of the TB bacteria can confirm the diagnosis within days.

A "Low–cost kit detects germs in just 5 minutes" has been reported as late as 2010[7]. A Taiwan scientist has invented the first low-cost and efficient test kit for identifying tuberculosis bacteria. The kit, which looks like those used for pregnancy tests, can establish whether samples taken from a suspected TB patient are positive or not in less than five minutes. Depending upon its reliability the kit can be useful in large scale screening surveys of suspected patients.

1.8 TREATMENT OF TUBERCULOSIS

Historically and until the discovery of antibiotics, the treatment of tuberculosis like that of other diseases was dominated by superstition. Fantastic theories about the treatment continued to prevail until the middle ages, apparently in disregard to the facts contained in the teachings of Hippocrates and Galen. These studies pointed out the importance of diet and personal hygiene, and avoidance of contact in the prevention and treatment of tuberculosis. The prevailing practice included priority to use of drugs designated mainly to relieve symptoms. Items such as garlic, tannin, mercury, arsenic, sulphur, calcium, iodides and gold were included in the treatment.

[7]The Times of India, March 30, 2010.

Preventive measures were rudimentary or irrelevant and apparently were given little importance. Even as late as the 17th and 18th centuries, little progress was made in this direction. With the exception of use of additional items such as cod liver oil and regular exercise to the existing treatment regimes, little was done to prevent tuberculosis. The following discussion is confined to the current procedures and medicine(s) used for the treatment of tuberculosis. However, methods used in the past from time to time for the treatment of tuberculosis are described in the chapter on the Historical Developments.

The availability of a spectrum of medications has made tuberculosis a curable disease. It may be noted that, with appropriate antibiotic treatment, TB can be cured in more than nine out of ten patients. However, certain points have to be kept in perspective while undertaking treatment. To begin with a difference between infection and disease has to be understood. Persons with TB infection but who do not have TB disease cannot spread the infection to other people. Therefore a person who has TB infection but does not have TB disease is not considered a case of TB. Such a person is often referred to as having latent TB infection (LTBI). This distinction is important because treatment options depend on whether a person has LTBI or an active status of TB disease. People with latent tuberculosis may be considered for treatment with a single anti-tubercular drug (isoniazid) to prevent the inactive disease from becoming active.

Further, it is important to bear in mind that a successful treatment of TB depends on close cooperation between the patient and doctor and other health care workers. Treatment usually combines several different antibiotic drugs which are given for at least six months, sometimes for as long as 12 months.

The most important aspect of present system of treatment is that patients must take their medicine on time every day during the entire period of treatment. Mid-way discontinuation of medicine(s) has got several serious health implications including development of drug resistant disease which may become incurable later. It has been noted that some TB patients stop taking their prescribed medicines because they start feeling better after only a couple of weeks of treatment. Unpleasant side effects of TB medicine(s) have also been cited as reasons for discontinuation of taking medicines regularly as required.

Chemotherapy

Following the discovery of streptomycin for treatment of tuberculosis in 1944 several drugs were added subsequently to cover the full range of infections. The anti-tubercular medications currently in use are:

- Isoniazid
- Pyrazinamide
- Rifampicin
- Ethambutol
- Cycloserine
- Para-Amino-Salicylic (PAS)
- Streptomycin
- Aminoglycosides (capreomycin, viomycin, kanamycin, and amikacin)
- Quinolones (levofloxin, ofloxacin, and ciprofloxacin).

Specific treatment in each case is determined by the physician based on:

- Patient's age, overall health, and medical history.
- Extent of the disease.
- Tolerance to specific medications, procedures and therapies.
- Expectations for the course of the disease.
- Need for short-term hospitalization.

Newer drugs and combination therapies are being studied by the Global Alliance for TB Drug Development in an effort to shorten treatment.

The three important properties of anti-TB drugs are: antibacterial activity, capacity to inhibit the development of resistance, and capacity to kill intracellular, persisting organisms. The initial combination of isoniazid, rifampin, pyrazinamide, and ethambutal provide effective TB treatment.

The bacilli responsible for most newly diagnosed and untreated cases of pulmonary tuberculosis are sensitive to three standard drugs, streptomycin, PAS and isoniazid. After the sensitivity has been established by testing bacilli cultured from sputum (requiring a few weeks, during which all three drugs are often given), treatment commonly continues with isoniazid (the most potent) accompanied by either of the two others. The underlying principle for giving a combination therapy is that it reduces the possibility of emergence of drug-resistant bacteria.

With the proper four-drug regimen, a rapid clinical improvement and a significant decrease in infectiousness is seen within a few weeks. After a month, the patients are generally without fever, feel well, and regain weight and strength. Coughing and sputum decrease and improvements in lesions are visible on the X-rays. Although bacteria may still be present in the smears, they become more and more difficult to culture and isolate. Patients are not infectious to others after one month of therapy.

The absence of radiological improvement in the first three months should be grounds for concern and indicate that a change in therapy may be needed. Patient adherence and the bacteria's drug sensitivity should be reevaluated. Relapses usually occur within six months of the end of treatment, and in most cases are due to poor patient adherence or inadequate treatment. Patient adherence must be monitored throughout treatment; through directly observed therapy (DOT), which should be the standard of care in every setting for all patients.

A study in India has shown that modern chemotherapy is so powerful that even ill-nourished overcrowded patients benefit; consequently mass chemotherapy for tuberculosis should probably be in the forefront of national policies. However, higher living standards (good housing and nutrition) may assist in reducing the spread of the disease in the community and so lower its incidence; health education of the patients and improved health consciousness of the public can also play a helpful role in control programmes.

Caution

If TB becomes active again in a previously treated patient, there is a high chance that the bacteria will become drug resistant. In this scenario current therapy should be suspended until multiple drugs are found to which the pathogen is fully sensitive. Anti-tubercular therapy can be resumed with the addition of these drugs to the original regimen. Some of the drugs that are used for resistant strains are:

- Ethionamide
- Cycloserine
- Capreomycin
- Kanamycin
- Streptomycin

Other Treatment Measures

Sanatorium stay and bed-rest have been virtually discarded from modern treatment regimens. Selective surgical procedures or local drainage of infected lesions are now restricted to a small minority of cases in which chemotherapy proves inadequate, or to drain the pus before start of therapy.

Duration of Treatment

Tuberculosis patients, according to WHO's guidelines[8], can be treated either by following an eight-month regimen or a six-month one. In the case of former regimen, all four antibiotics are given for the first two months, and two drugs for the remaining six months. Rifampicin is not one of the drugs given during the remaining six months. This was the option given to resource-poor countries and where DOTS implementation was difficult. By contrast, in the case of the latter regimen, all the four drugs are administered for the first two months, and rifampicin and another antibiotic for the remaining four months. The medicines can be given either daily or thrice a week (intermittent dosing schedule) during the entire course of the therapy. The research has shown that there was increased risk of poor treatment outcomes and drug resistance when rifampicin was not given throughout the six-month therapy period and when it was given only during the first two months in the case of the eight-month regimen.

India and China are the only two countries that have opted for thrice a week regimen during the six-month regimen. Most

---

[8]The Hindu, New Delhi, September 17, 2009.

developed countries have gone in for the daily regimen. India has been facing much criticism for treating patients by using a different regimen, especially since it has a huge disease burden. China is only other country that follows the same regimen as India. There are several reasons for choosing the thrice-a-week regimen. These include: convenience, reduced cost by more than half, and less adverse reactions. It also enables the implementation of DOTS.

Earlier WHO had changed the treatment guidelines for newly diagnosed untreated patients from six months to eight months to be used in the 24–high-incidence countries. According to the study such a change was not required. Now WHO recommends only the six-month (rifampicin throughout) regimen, and the eight-month regimen will no longer be recommended.

The minimum duration of treatment is six months. Depending on the severity of the disease the doctor will decide whether to give medicines daily or intermittently. The duration of treatment, however, in some cases might be extended to a maximum of nine months or more.

To avoid relapse or developing into a resistant form of disease, the instructions given by the doctor about taking the medicine should be strictly adhered to. Most relapses occur when patients begin to feel better and stop medications against medical advice. Such patients can then become infectious to other people.

Completion of Treatment

If patients do not take all their medicines the way their doctor tells them, they can become sick again and spread TB to their friends and family. Additionally, when patients do not take all the drugs the doctor has prescribed or skip times when they are supposed to take them, the TB bacteria learn to outwit the TB antibiotics, and soon those medications no longer work against the disease. If this happens, the person now has resistant TB infection. Some patients have disease that is resistant to two or more drugs. This is called multidrug-resistant TB or

MDR-TB because the TB germ, *M. tuberculosis* resists eradication with more than one drug. This form of TB is much more difficult to cure.

Tuberculosis and Pregnancy

TB can occur in pregnancy, as it is an infectious disease. In such cases, however, the disease poses a diagnostic challenge[9]. TB and pregnancy are two different kinds of stresses that women experience. Their simultaneous occurrence would result in so much strain that it tends to impact the growing foetus as well. TB can affect organs and TB of certain organs poses a diagnostic challenge. Since it is an infectious disease, late diagnosis and non-diagnosis can affect both the baby and the mother. In the mother, the disease can become extensive and spread to the baby resulting in a condition called congenital TB.

TB is mainly diagnosed by bacteriology and X-rays. During pregnancy, X-rays have to be taken carefully as they are harmful to the foetus. If the X-ray is essential, the abdomen should be covered with a metal shield. It is a precaution all concerned including the mother should observe when asked to take X-rays during pregnancy. Getting a bacteriological diagnosis is still more difficult, as they cannot cough to bring out sputum. Even in those who give sputum the chances of picking up bacilli is only 30 per cent.

The treatment regimen is the same as that for any other TB patient. However, there may be some difference in scheduling of different drugs. It depends on the stage at which the diagnosis is made. For example, if the diagnosis is made in the first two months, the priority will be to treat TB rather than maintaining pregnancy. At this point, when organogenesis occurs, the effect of drugs on the foetus is debatable. On the contrary, when diagnosis is made in the second or third trimester all the drugs can be given safely as none of the drugs cross the placenta. This will prevent extension of the disease in the mother and also the spread to the baby.

---

[9]Diagnostic challenge, The Hindu, New Delhi, March 22, 2009.

1.9 DRUG-RESISTANT TB

Drug-resistance

With appropriate antibiotic therapy available today, TB is curable. However, in recent years drug-resistant cases of the disease have increased dramatically. The resistance results when antibiotics used to combat it are carelessly administered by poorly trained doctors or patients don't take their full course of medication consistently for the six to 12 months necessary to destroy all vestiges of *M. tuberculosis*. It may also develop when patients are treated with too few drugs or with inadequate doses. Rather than being killed by the drugs, the bacterium that causes TB mutates and the microbe builds up resistance to them.

TB Re-treatment Raises Drug-resistance Risk[10]

An alarming 20% of the people availing re-treatment of tuberculosis are at the risk of developing multidrug resistance TB in India. According to the Global Health Advocates, of the 196,000 people who registered themselves for re-treatment for TB in 2004, 39,000 showed drug-resistance.

There are four main reasons why patients stop medication, leading to drug resistance. These are: migration and/or homeless status, alcohol and drug dependency, apparent disappearance of symptoms after taking medicine for a month or two, and violent side-effects, generally in that order of occurrence. In addition, stigma against TB continues to be an issue that comes in the way of effective treatment and leads a patient to default. Interaction between poverty on the one hand and several of these factors on the other can seriously impact the rise in default rate.

Multidrug Resistant TB

Particularly alarming is the increase in the number of people with multidrug-resistant TB (MDR-TB), caused by *M. tuberculosis* strains resistant to two or more most potent first

[10]Kounteya Sinha, Times of India, New Delhi, March 27, 2007.

line anti-tuberculosis drugs, namely isoniazid (INH) and rifampicin (RMP). This form of TB is much more difficult to cure. Isolates that are resistant to any other combination of anti-TB drugs but not to INH and RMP are not classed as MDR-TB.

Even with treatment, the death rate for MDR-TB patients is 40 to 60 percent, the same as for TB patients who receive no treatment. For people co-infected with HIV and MDR-TB, the death rate may be as high as 80 percent. The time from diagnosis to death for some patients with MDR-TB and HIV may be only months as they are sometimes left with no treatment options.

It is unusual for MDR-TB to spread from person to person, except in the context of weakened immune system as those with HIV or some other cause of immune suppression. Outbreaks among normal healthy people do occur, but is uncommon. About a third of the 35 countries surveyed in 1997 showed rates above 2% for MDR-TB. The highest rates were in the former USSR, the Baltic states, Argentina, India and China, and were associated with poor or failing national tuberculosis control programmes.

Prevention of MDR TB

In the Indian context, as elsewhere, prevention of MDR-TB should be given highest priority. To achieve this we need to step up awareness, case detection and IEC activities. Patients have to be informed about the cost and time effectiveness of going through the entire course of medication as advised. It should be stressed on the beneficiaries (patients and relatives) that the entire course of first line treatment under directly observed treatment short-course (DOTS) where drugs have to be taken thrice a week lasts between six and nine months and costs about Rs. 2000 should be adhered to. By contrast, the course of second line drugs takes two years has more side-effects and costs about Rs. 2 lakh. Additionally, more drugs have to be taken daily.

In the initial phase of the DOTS programme, there was a blitz in the media. Facts about TB and DOTS treatment were being disseminated widely. Now, this has reached a kind of stagnation. The staff shortage in TB control posts in many States affects the programme adversely. As a result the new entrants, including the field staff and DOTS providers, are not getting enough training and motivation. The entire programme including case detection and cure rate suffers. The international Stop TB Partnership also advocates that communities can stop TB by sharing information on how to prevent it. Awareness generation is also said to have a major role to play in reducing stigma and therefore, discrimination. Further, the national programme in India considered that the most effective means of preventing further resistance was by maintaining and improving the quality of treatment and, more importantly promoting rational use of anti-TB drugs.

Treatment of MDR TB

Treatment for MDR-TB often requires the use of special TB drugs, all of which can produce serious side effects. To cure MDR-TB, patients may have to take several antibiotics, at least three to which the bacteria still respond, every day for up to two years. However, even with this treatment, between four and six out of ten patients with MDR-TB will die, which is the same as for patients with normal TB who do not receive treatment. Economically, dealing with MDR TB is a big blow for the programme. Medicines for drug resistant TB are highly expensive—50 to 200 times higher than those for simple form of tuberculosis.

Of the alternate regimens available currently, the specific treatment, like that in the case of fully sensitive TB, is determined by the physician based on patient's:

- Age, overall health, and medical history.
- Extent of the disease.
- Tolerance for specific medications, procedures, or therapies.
- Expectations for the course of the disease.
- Opinion or preference.
- Short-term hospitalization
- Medications

Treatment may last for many months. However, once the treatment begins, the patient begins to feel well very soon. The patient is not usually contagious once treatment begins, provided that treatment is carried through to the end, as prescribed by a physician.

Extreme Drug-resistant TB (XDR-TB)[11]

A virulent strain of tuberculosis resistant to most available drugs (XDR-TB) is surfacing around the globe, raising fears of a pandemic that could devastate efforts to contain TB and prove deadly to people with immune-deficiency diseases such as HIV-AIDS. It is caused by bacteria that is resistant to the most effective anti-TB drugs and has emerged from the mismanagement of multidrug-resistant TB (MDR-TB). XDR-TB is defined as TB that has developed resistance to at least rifampicin and isoniazid (MDR-TB), as well as to any member of the quinolone family and at least one of the following second-line anti-TB injectable drugs: kanamycin, capreomycin, or amikacin. This definition of XDR-TB agreed by the WHO Global Task Force on XDR-TB in October 2006 supersedes the earlier definition of XDR-TB as MDR-TB that was also resistant to three or more of the six classes of second-line drugs. Further, with restricted treatment options, the strain is likely to jeopardize the major gains made in TB control and progress on reducing TB deaths among people living with HIV/AIDS. It is therefore vital that TB control is managed properly and new tools developed to prevent, treat and diagnose the disease.

1.10 ROLE OF RESEARCH IN THE FIGHT AGAINST TB

Institutions worldwide continue in their endeavour to better understand how *M. tuberculosis* infects and causes disease in humans and also how the human immune system responds to it. This research will help to develop new tools to diagnose TB, find better vaccines, and new medicines against TB. Below are some important advances that have been made in TB research.

[11]The Tribune, New Delhi, May 5, 2007 by arrangement with LA – Times Washington Post.

Diagnosis: Potential new tests to speed the diagnosis of TB from four weeks to two days; differences found in the DNA of *M. tuberculosis* and the bacterium used in the BCG vaccine may lead to a test to tell the difference between people who really have TB and those who only react to previous BCG vaccination.

Treatment: Discovery of the molecules responsible for drug resistance, knowledge that will help doctors quickly select the best treatments for their patients; a new drug under study can be taken less often to help patients comply with their treatment regimen.

In a landmark study that could provide new pathways for tuberculosis (TB) therapy, Indian scientists have unlocked the secret formula that the TB bacterium uses to survive inside the human body[12]. This has the potential to create a TB therapy free from antibiotics-based drugs and consequently could be a valuable tool in the fight against antibiotic resistant TB.

Cure for Extreme TB Strain Found[13]

American scientists have found that a combination of two FDA-approved drugs Clavulanate and Meropenem, meant for fighting other bacterial infections like *E. coli*, completely blocked the growth of 13 strains of XDR TB which were isolated in the lab. Scientists successfully killed all XDR TB bacteria in less than two weeks time.

According to scientists from Albert Einstein College of Medicine in New York and National Institute of Allergy and Infectious Diseases (NIAID), the drugs worked in tandem—while one brought down the guard of the TB bacteria by inhibiting the enzyme that normally shields it from antibiotics, the other killed it. The entire discovery happened by chance when after three years of lab research, Clavulanate was found to be highly effective in inhibiting the crucial enzyme that shielded TB bacteria while Meropenem was highly effective in killing the TB organism completely. Normally, it takes two years of continuous therapy to treat drug resistant TB strains. However, if the new combination works in humans, it will be

[12]India unlocks TB germ secrets, The Hindustan Times, March 5, 2010.
[13]Times of India, New Delhi, April 8, 2009.

able to completely eliminate the organism within two weeks time. Phase II clinical trials on humans are now being planned simultaneously in South Korea and South Africa.

Vaccines: More than 90 vaccine candidates have been developed and tested in animals.

Training: An innovative telemedicine programme and grassroot health promotion programmes can extend training and education to health workers and physicians working in remote areas and under resource constraint situations. In this regard a global TB research agenda developed by NIAID is relevant. For desired impact it will require a concerted global collaborations with sister agencies and other organizations with similar goals such as the Global Alliance for TB Drug Development and the STOP TB initiative, as well as partnerships with governments and scientists from countries where the burden of tuberculosis is greatest.

Breakthrough in TB Control[14]

Indian scientists have achieved a major technological breakthrough in the treatment of tuberculosis. The new technology developed and patented by BV Patel Pharma-ceutical Education and Research Development (PERD) Centre promises, for the first time in 14 years, a solution to drug-resistant TB that is hampering the National TB Control programme.

The new anti-TB drug formulation (single capsule) can enhance treatment efficiency by 30 per cent and reduce TB treatment period by half. It does away with gross treatment inefficacies witnessed in the presently marketed fixed dose two-drug combination of Rifampicin and Isoniazid being administered to TB patients because the drugs chemically react in the patient's stomach and neutralise each other. This reaction reduces efficacy by 30 per cent and more in tropical climates because of which treatment remains sub-optimal and takes longer time, allowing pathogenic bacteria to develop immunity to drugs. This is the primary cause behind poor progress of TB Control Programme.

---

[14]The Tribune, New Delhi, June 7, 2010.

The new compartmentalised formulation to separate the two TB drugs in the capsule developed at PERD works by segregating Rifampicin and Isoniazid in the capsule and the patient's body. Since the two drugs under new formulation do not see each other and therefore do not react, the efficacy of the treatment is enhanced by 30 per cent and the treatment period is reduced by half. The formulation is expected to work for all types of TB.

In the new formulation Rifampicin is retained in the stomach for six hours before being absorbed from the stomach while Isoniazid is technologically prevented (though enteric coating) from dissolving in the stomach. The latter drug goes past the stomach and dissolves only on reaching the alkaline atmosphere of intestines. This separation solves the old problem. Funded by the Department of Biotechnology and Union Ministry of Chemicals, the project is at an advanced stage of trials. The AIIMS and PERD Centre will take up final comparative trials involving old and new drug formulations on TB patients before general use.

Scientists Decode TB Enzyme, to make New Drugs[15]

Decoding of the unique structure and mechanism of a tuberculosis enzyme by scientists at Maryland University College of Chemical and Life Sciences, US, recently has paved the way for development of new drugs to combat active and latent tuberculosis infections.

The development of new TB drugs has become urgent, as strains of TB resistant to all major anti-TB drugs have emerged worldwide.

TB Treatment to take just 2 Months[16]

A new regimen of treatment developed at the Tuberculosis Research Centre (TRC), Chennai can help cure the disease in two months, instead of six months. This will be of great advantage over the existing protocol and will certainly reduce

[15]Times of India, New Delhi, March 28, 2009.

[16]Times of India, New Delhi, March 28, 2009.

drop-out rates and possibly side-effects. Here a drug has been added to the existing four-drug regimen to make it more effective. Under the present system at DOTS, isoniazid, rifampicin, pyrazinamide and ethambutol are administered for two months and isoniazid and rifampicin are given for four months. The patient is considered cured after six months. Now, moxiflocin has been added to reduce the treatment period. The initial results show that the new regimen has a great potential for treating multidrug resistant TB.

Drug that makes TB Germs Self-Destruct Raises Hope of Cure[17]

Australian scientists at Sydney's Centenary Institute recently developed a drug which could essentially cure tuberculosis at its non-infectious stage. This drug could be heralded as the first major breakthrough on the disease in 50 years. This research which is looking at the genetics of TB, when brought to utilization stage, has the potential for saving millions of lives around the world. The researchers investigated a protein essential for survival of TB bacteria and successfully developed a drug that would inhibit this protein. The work on identifying the full extent of the drug's potential is in progress. This finding has shown the way for the first time in history that dormant or asymptomatic, non-infectious TB can be treated. This will potentially stem a deadly tide of infection because the available antibiotics used to fight TB are effective only against active TB which manifests only in one of ten inactive cases.

[17]Times of India, New Delhi, March 25, 2010, The Hindu, New Delhi, March 25, 2010.

2

Historical Developments

2.1 INTRODUCTION

Tuberculosis is one of the most ancient diseases in the world. Based on a number of archeological researches, the occurrence of disease has been noted in several countries at various times. However, lack of communications tended to limit its world spread, and consequently large areas were free from it until exposed to contacts with infected, economically more developed populations. Previously isolated, primitive communities with little inbuilt immunity for the disease proved to be virgin soil for the spread of tuberculosis. The mortality rose from nil to appalling figures and the disease went through an acute course. The severity of the epidemics was enhanced by factors usually associated with bad living conditions. In due course of time the mortality declined and other factors gradually changed and the disease assumed a more chronic pattern. The improvement was considered to be due to a combination of generic selection and improved living standards.

In many industrialized or semi-industrialized countries the death rate due to tuberculosis increased during the period of their initial industrialization and increasing urbanization in the 18th and 19th century when such areas experienced substantial over-crowding, bad working conditions and other environmental factors conducive to the spread of infection. The general tendency for the mortality was to attain a peak and then decline gradually to a low level eventually. Sometimes the trend was interrupted by national catastrophes such as war. To illustrate we may note that in England and Wales the death rate due to tuberculosis was estimated to have risen from its level in the early 18th century to a peak of over 1,000 per 100,000 persons in 1780-1800, followed by a steady decline, interrupted by sharp rises in 1914-18 and 1939-41. The decline was much accelerated after the introduction of chemotherapy in 1948-52; the death rate of 7.5 per 100,000 persons in 1960 was about one-fifth of that in 1950 (36.4), the fall being greatest in the younger age groups.

Tuberculosis which was responsible for 20% of deaths in London in the 1600s, over 30% of deaths in Paris in the 1800s has attained the status of a global emergency today according to the World Health Organization.

This chapter briefly describes the historical developments from the oldest known or believed evidence to the present about the nomenclature, prevalence and treatment of tuberculosis. Various aliases of the disease are presented in Section 2.2. The following three sections respectively deal with developments along the time scale. While the ancient history of tuberculosis covers the period from beginning of the civilization to the fall of Roman Empire (Section 2.3), the medieval period covers the developments thereafter and up to the end of 19th century (Section 2.4). The developments that took place during the 20th century and later are covered in Section 2.5. The chapter covers the historical developments in the context of India in Section 2.6.

2.2 ALIASES OF TUBERCULOSIS

Depending on the nature of the disease, the place and time, tuberculosis has been known under a variety of names during the course of history. It has often been a difficult disease to diagnose and has been confused with many other diseases. The disease has been also known under other names, such as phthisis, Scrofula, tabes, bronchitis, and inflammation of the lungs, hectic fever, gastric fever, and lupus. It was also known as the great white plague or "consumption". The word consumption is employed in the Bible to translate Schache-pheth, which is also the Modern Hebrew word for tuberculosis. Although tuberculosis can attack the whole body, it is frequently known more for its damage to the lungs (Table 2.1). These names described different forms or aspects of the disease. The physicians of antiquity, in India, Greece and Rome, provided accurate description of the symptoms of phthisis and scrofula. The "Great White Plague" which started in Europe in the 1600's and continued for 200 years was Tuberculosis. Other names throughout history for tuberculosis are Phthisis (from the Greek word to waste away), scrofula (swellings of the lymph nodes of the neck), consumption (progressive wasting away of the body) and TB (the presence or products of the tubercle bacillus).

These diseases were considered largely the result of an inherent constitutional trait, and if contact was considered dangerous, that was in the sense of, say, a sympathetic vibration. Table 2.1 gives a run of various names that have been given to the disease from time to time. However, the most common name for the disease as known today (tuberculosis) came after the discovery of the tubercles found in infected patients by Dr. Sylvius, better known as Franciscus de la Boe, in 1679.

Table 2.1: Various names given to tuberculosis in the past

Name of Disease	*Disease/Symptoms*
Phthisis and phthisis pulmonalis	It is the Greek name for consumption. Originally identified by Hippocrates in 460BC, it was the most widespread disease of the times and was almost always fatal. It was associated with chronic wasting away.
King's Evil	Tuberculosis of the lymph glands and neck was known as King's Evil because of the belief in medieval times that newly crowned Kings of England and France had the powers to heal TB with their touch.
Koch's Disease	This name was given after Robert Koch who discovered the tuberculosis bacilli.

Contd...

Table 2.1: Various names given to tuberculosis in the past (*Contd...*)

Name of Disease	*Disease/Symptoms*
Lung Sickness	Tuberculosis signified this disease because of its involvement with lungs.
Lupus vulgaris	The common wolf–Tuberculosis of the skin.
Mesenteric disease	This term stood for tuberculosis of the abdominal lymph glands. It was caused by consumption of milk from cows infected with TB. The milk generally consumed today is pasteurized and therefore this form of the disease is no longer prevalent.
Miliary TB	This name derives from the fact that X-ray lesions look like millet seeds.
Consumption	Tuberculosis seemed to consume people from within with its symptoms of bloody cough, fever, pallor, and long relentless wasting.
Pott's disease	Tuberculosis infection of the spine, TB of the bone with characteristic vertebra fusion and deformity of the spine.
Prosector's wart	A kind of TB of the skin, transmitted by contact with contaminated cadavers, to anatomists, surgeons, butchers, etc.
Scrofula	Tuberculosis of the lymph glands (swollen glands of the neck).
Tabes mesenterica	TB of the abdomen
TB	Short for tuberculosis and also for Tubercle Bacillus.
White Plague	Tuberculosis TB sufferers appear markedly pale.
White swelling	Tuberculosis infection of the bones.

2.3 ANCIENT HISTORY OF TUBERCULOSIS

(From beginning of civilization to the fall of Roman Empire in AD 476)

The tuberculosis germ may be as old as the Earth itself. Probably it survived in the primeval mud in the very early days. Among the humans also it has possibly been present since antiquity. The origins of the disease are in the first domestication of cattle. The germ first infected animals-possibly inhaled or ingested from the soil. *M. bovis* had been causing TB in animal kingdom long before invading humanity. It affects many kinds of animals including cows, birds, fish and reptiles.

Several evidences suggest that following the domestication of animals during 8000–4000 BC, the human population suffered from infection by *M. bovis*, possibly through the animal's flesh and milk injestation. This shows that the disease has been there with us for a long time now. A number of archeological findings have confirmed this prevalence in the past around 5000–1000 BC. The earliest evidence of TB in humans as detected from a neolithic grave near Heidleberg, Germany, puts the date back to 5000 BC. Examinations of the spines of mummies and of tomb paintings from 4000 BC confirm that TB was a common disease in Egypt. Mummies from 3000–2400 BC have shown evidence of TB of the spines. Similar findings were reported from skeletal remains in Italy from dates around the same time which also confirmed the prevalence of TB of the spine. References cite that prehistoric humans had TB around 4000 BC. Indications of lung scarring identical to that of modern-day TB sufferers in preserved bodies (such as mummies) suggests that TB was present in The Americas from about 2000 BC.

Evidence of TB appears in Biblical scripture, in Chinese literature dating back to around 4000 BC, and in religious books in India around 2000 BC. References to the disease are found in India during the Vedic period (1800 BC – 600 BC) as contained in Vedas and Ayurvedic Samhitas. It got mentioned in the works of Ancient *Ayurvedic* System of medicines practised by *Sushrutha, Charaka* and others around 2500 BC. In this system all the diseases (including tuberculosis) were considered to result due to imbalance among three *dosas* (defects) of the body. These are: *Vata* (combination of Air and Earth), *Pitta* (Fire) and *Kapha* (Water and Earth). It is not clear whether the infectious nature of the disease was recognized by the ancient system. In ancient Greece Hippocrates mentions TB around 400 BC. Aristotle talked about "phthisis and its cure" around 350 BC.

It is believed that TB was prevalent around 2500–1500 BC in mainland Europe. However, the earliest evidence of the disease in Britain comes from graves dating back to Roman occupation (55 BC–800 AD).

It is possible that *M. bovis* was likely pathogan in human TB until 1000 BC. After 1000 BC widespread pulmonary TB emerged. In fact *M. tuberculosis* probably is an evolved, specialized form of *M. bovis* developed among milk-drinking Indo- Europeans who then spread the disease during their migration into Western - Europe and Eurasia. By the 1st millennium BC, *M.tb* causing pulmonary TB had spread throughout the known world. Earliest tangible record of pulmonary TB was discovered between 668 BC to 626 BC. The classic TB signs cough expectoration, hemoptysis, wasting of the body, were well recognized. The earliest written evidence of pulmonary TB was from the library of the Assyrian King Assur Baninpal (668–626 BC). Table 2.2 provides a timeline for various evidences which suggest the prevalence of tuberculosis during the prehistoric period.

The term "phthisis", consumption, appeared first in Greek literature. Around 460 BCE, Hippocrates identified phthisis as the most widespread disease of the times, and noted that it was almost always fatal. Due to common phthisis-related fatalities, he wrote something no doctor would dare write today. He warned his colleagues against visiting TB patients in late stages of the disease, because their inevitable deaths might damage the reputations of the attending physicians.

Tuberculosis has been one of the major causes of mortality for thousands of years. The severity was compounded by widespread enabling conditions such as overcrowding, sanitation issues, malnutrition, and a lack of knowledge surrounding the disease.

Table 2.2: Timeline for evidence of prevalence of tuberculosis in human population during prehistoric period

8000BC–4000 BC	Evidence of human infection by *M. bovis* after the domestication of animals.
5000 BC–1000 BC	Evidence of spinal tuberculosis (Pott disease).
5000 BC	Examination of Neolithic graves near Heidleberg, Germany, showed evidence of TB.
4000 BC–2400 BC	Chinese literature dating back to 4000 BC mentions about tuberculosis. Examination of fragments of spinal column of Egyptian mummies showed evidence of Pott's disease (tuberculosis) as common disease in Egypt. Tuberculosis infection was also detected from mummies belonging to Early Bronze Age from Babe dh-Dhra, Jordon.
2500 BC–1500 BC	Occurrence of TB was established in mainland Europe.
1800 BC–600 BC	Reference to the tuberculosis in India during the Vedic Period.
1000 BC	Possible starting time for emergence of pulmonary tuberculosis.
668 BC – 626 BC	Earliest tangible record of pulmonary tuberculosis obtained from the library of the Assyrian King Assur Baninpal.
460 BC	Hippocrates identified phthisis (earlier name of TB) as the most widespread disease of the times and noted that it was almost always fatal. He, even as a doctor, warned his collegues against visiting TB patients in late stages of the disease, mainly to protect the reputation of the doctors.
350 BC	Aristotle's writings mention the disease "phthisis" and its cure
55 BC – 800 AD	Evidence of TB from graves in UK under Roman occupation.
200 AD	Roman doctor Claudius Galen observed that consumption was incurable and recommended a treatment regimen which included living in fresh air, plenty of rest and good diet.

2.4 MEDIEVAL HISTORY OF TUBERCULOSIS

(Fall of Roman Empire to the end of 19th century)

Many early attempts at treatment can be found throughout the world. Greeks believed cutting off cool air eventuated in a burning-up of the tissues of the body. The Romans put great importance on the diet. The Hebrews appear to have been exposed to TB for many years, and made a number of attempts to control the disease from diet to the destruction of clothing. Early reported "cures" from physicians included warm sea air, milk from pregnant women, seaweed placed under the pillow, cold baths and deep breathing. Most of these proved to be fruitless, and it would be many years before any real cures could be found. Many people , according to a number of ancient literatures, including the Bible, believed that the disease was a form of punishment. By 1650 consumption was the leading cause of mortality and it became a reference in some of Shakespeare's plays, one of the consumptive lovers, in "Much Ado About Nothing", as well as scrofula in Macbeth.

Most of the medieval period did not see much activity in extending our understanding about tuberculosis. However, the presence of TB was detected in 11th century mummies of Pre-Colombian period in Peru. Until late in the 20th century it was thought that Columbus brought TB to the new world in 1492. The change came when scientists reported in 1994 that they had identified TB bacterium DNA in the mummified remains of a woman who died in the America 500 years before Columbus set sail for the New World. This confirmed the presence of tuberculosis in Latin America even before the colonization by the Europeans and provided a setback to somewhat prevalent notion at the time that migration of Europeans played a role in the spread of the disease. Nothing much was found until the middle of the 16th century when in 1546 Fracastorio suggested that a living contagion was involved in the tuberculosis. About the same time Girolamo Tracastoro wrote the book *De Morbis Contagionis* which described the contagious nature of tuberculosis. It even suggested that bed sheets and clothing of patients could contain contagious particles.

By the mid 17th century, one in five deaths in London—as recorded in the Bills of Mortality—were due to TB (consumption). TB soon became an epidemic in Britain and major cities in the USA and Europe. It was known as the "White Plague". By the turn of the 19th century, the estimation of world wide TB death rate was high enough to generate a fear that by the end of the 19th century, European population might be destroyed. London and New York were two of the worst affected cities.

Despite the significant level of understanding about the etiology of consumption, which had already initiated prevention and a break in the chain of infection, there was little progress towards finding a cure for the disease. Only after the advances in scientific knowledge of the disease in the mid-19 century backed with solid evidence that it could heal, technology for rational treatment and prevention of tuberculosis could begin to emerge. Rest and plentiful diet became the regimen of choice. Despite Koch's discovery in 1882 the high hopes of specific cure of tuberculosis by chemical agents were unfulfilled. This gap occasioned the establishment and expansion of scope of sanatoria for treatment of tuberculosis-both pulmonary and other types, bed-rest and fresh air being the principles underlying both, and sun light playing an important role in the latter.

Exact pathological and anatomical descriptions of the disease, however, began to appear in the seventeenth century. In his *Opera Medica* of 1679, Sylvius was the first to identify actual tubercles showing a consistent and characteristic change in the lungs and other areas of consumptive patients. He also described their progression to abscesses and cavities. Manget described the pathological features of miliary tuberculosis in 1702. The earliest references to the infectious nature of the disease appear in seventeenth century Italian medical literature. An edict issued by the Republic of Lucca in 1699 states that, "henceforth, human health should no longer be endangered by objects remaining after the death of a consumptive. The names of the deceased should be reported to the authorities, and measures undertaken for disinfection".

In 1720, the English physician Benjamin Marten was the first to conjecture, in his publication, *A New Theory of Consumption*, that TB could be caused by "wonderfully minute living creatures," which, after gaining a foothold in the body, could generate the lesions and symptoms of the disease. He stated, moreover, "It may be therefore very likely that by an habitual lying in the same bed with a consumptive patient, constantly eating and drinking with him, or by very frequently conversing so nearly as to draw in part of the breath he emits from the lungs, a consumption may be caught by a sound person. I imagine that slightly conversing with consumptive patients is seldom or never sufficient to catch the disease". For the early eighteenth century, Dr. Marten's writings display a great degree of epidemiological insight.

The introduction of the sanatorium cure was the first real and significant step towards curing tuberculosis. The initiative was based on the findings of an interesting research project where Hermann Brehmer, a Silesian botany student suffering from TB, was instructed by his doctor to seek out a healthier climate. Accordingly he travelled to the Himalayan mountains where he could pursue his botanical studies while trying to rid himself of the disease. He returned home cured and began to study medicine. In 1854, he presented his doctoral dissertation entitled *Tuberculosis is a Curable Disease*. In the same year, he built a house in the middle of a pine forest in Gorbersdorf, where he combined botanical research with a search to find a cure for tuberculosis. In this establishment sick patients were given much wholesome food and, in the midst of fir trees, they were exposed to continuous fresh air in plenty available on their balconies. This setup became the blueprint for the most modern way to fight the disease and subsequent development of sanatoria system, a powerful weapon in the battle against an insidious opponent. This idea was soon followed by sanatoria being developed in USA. In UK where, in the second half of the nineteenth century, many consumption patients were nursed (and died) in the poor law institutions the pressure was exerted now for opening of sanatoria in England and Wales. The sanatoria provided medical care for almost 100 years and became one of the most remarkable and unique ways of medical care in history.

Since, TB displayed the variety of symptoms, it could be identified as a unified disease only by as late as the 1820s. It was named tuberculosis by J L Schönlein only in 1839. The use of environmental factors to cure following the findings about their role, the sanitoria movement began to gain momentum. Over a period of about seven years from 1838 to 1845, Dr. John Croghan, the owner of Mammoth Cave, brought a number of tuberculosis sufferers into the cave in hopes of curing the disease with the constant temperature and purity of the cave air. However, the first TB sanatorium opened in 1859 in Poland, a good five years after the presentation of the dissertation by Hermann Brehmer. It was followed by another one in the United States in 1885. New advances followed in rapid succession. In 1865, the French military doctor, Jean-Antoine Villemin single-handedly demonstrated that consumption could be passed from humans to cattle and from cattle to rabbits. On the basis of this revolutionary evidence, he postulated a specific microorganism as the cause of the disease, finally laying to rest the centuries-old belief that consumption arose spontaneously in each affected organism.

The measures available to doctors were still modest. Improving social and sanitary conditions, and ensuring adequate nutrition were all that could be done to strengthen the body's defenses against the TB bacillus. Thousands of sanatoria, to be found throughout Europe and the United States at that time, provided a dual function: they isolated the sick, the source of infection, from the general population, while the enforced rest, together with a proper diet and the well-regulated hospital life assisted the healing processes.

These efforts were reinforced by the observation of the Italian Forlanini, who in 1890 found that collapsing the lungs had a positive effect on the recovery from tuberculosis. Subsequently, with the introduction of artificial pneumothorax and surgical methods to reduce the lung volume, the depressing era of helplessness in the face of advanced TB was thought to be over, and that of active therapy had begun.

Mycobacterium tuberculosis, the bacillus that causes tuberculosis, was finally and successfully described on March

24, 1882 by Robert Koch, a German bacteriologist. The isolation of the infectious agent known as tuberculosis bacteria or tubercle bacilli was the first real breakthrough in understanding tuberculosis for which Koch was awarded the Nobel Prize in physiology or medicine in 1905 for this discovery. Robert Koch discovered a staining technique that enabled him to see Mycobacterium tuberculosis. What excited the world was not so much the scientific brilliance of Koch's discovery, but the accompanying certainty that heralded the beginning of the fight against humanity's deadliest enemy. Koch did not believe that bovine (cattle) and human tuberculosis were similar, which held back the recognition of infected milk as a source of infection. Later, this source was eliminated by pasteurization. Koch announced a glycerine extract of the tubercle bacilli as a "remedy" for tuberculosis in 1890, calling it tuberculin. It was not effective, but was later adapted by von Pirquet for a test for pre-symptomatic tuberculosis.

A further significant advance came in 1895 when Wilhelm Konrad von Rontgen discovered the radiation that would later bear his name. With this development the progress and severity of a patient's disease could be accurately followed and reviewed.

TB in America during the colonial period was accepted as a scourge of humanity that was common to the poor and rich alike. The first available mortality figures from Massachusetts in 1796 indicated 300 deaths per 100,000 persons. The peak mortality figure reached in New England was 1,600 per 100,000 in 1800. With the industrial development, the epidemic traveled to the Midwest in 1840 and to the West in 1880. The American Indians and Alaskans were the last American populations to become effected by the TB epidemic. At the turn of the century it was estimated that 10% of all deaths in the United States were due to TB.

In 1886, Edward Livingston Trudeau a physician who recovered from TB, started the sanatorium movement in the United States at Saranac Lake, New York. He based it on the European model of strict supervision in providing fresh air and sunshine, bed rest, and nutritious foods. As infection control measures took hold in large urban centers of the country, TB patients who could not be treated in local dispensaries were removed from the general population and placed into sanatoria. By 1938 there were more than 700 sanatoria throughout the US, yet the number of patients outnumbered the beds available.

In 1892, Dr. Herman Biggs of New York started mandatory reporting of TB cases. He thought that we should:

- Educate the public of the dangers that the disease posed to the person and his/her contacts.
- Properly dispose of and immediately destroy sputum or the "discharges from the lungs" of the individuals with disease.
- Have all physicians of pulmonary cases report such cases to the health department.
- Have health inspectors visit the families where TB exists and deliver proper literature and take specific measures to disinfect the areas as may be required.
- Obtain and submit sputum specimens to the laboratory for analysis.
- Create a consumptive hospital to care for indigent patients.

The board adopted most of the recommendations made by Biggs, including the creation of the Consumptive Hospital. These recommendations created a storm of controversy among the medical community. Many private doctors objected to the mandatory reporting, believing that it violated physician-patient confidentiality. Because of the resistance from the medical community, reporting practices were not fully implemented for several years. In the end, Biggs' recommendations to the Board and their implementation in New York City created the model for TB control programme that was emulated by other health departments across the country and laid the groundwork for a campaign called the "War on Consumption".

By 1889 in the USA, the National Tuberculosis Association fully realized that TB was distinctly preventable and that it was not directly inherited. The Association set out to educate the community at large. The idea was followed by France and

Germany in 1892 and the Dutch in 1897. A committee, named The National Association for the Prevention of Tuberculosis or NAPT, was formed. NAPT books for educating people about bad food, bad air and unhealthy drinking water were provided to members of the community. People were advised against overcrowding in the home, overworking and overstraining themselves. The NAPT could only advise and they had no real powers to improve city dwellers and tackle poverty. The UK soon followed the example set by the NAPT. The International Union against Tuberculosis was founded in 1902 with its offices based in Berlin. This office closed during the First World War but re-opened in Geneva in 1920. The International Union monitored the progress of the Institutions and encouraged a system of TB control throughout Europe.

Tuberculosis caused the most widespread public concern in the 19th and early 20th centuries as the endemic disease of the urban poor. The disease accounted for one in four deaths in England in 1815 and one in six deaths in France in, as late as, 1918. After the establishment in the 1880s that TB was contagious, it was made a notifiable disease in Britain; there were campaigns to stop spitting in public places, and the infected poor were "encouraged" to enter sanatoria that rather resembled prisons. Whatever the purported benefits of the fresh air and labour in the sanatoria, 75% of those who entered were dead within five years.

In the United States, concern about the spread of tuberculosis played a role in the movement to prohibit public spitting except into spittoons.

In Europe, deaths from TB fell from 500 out of 100,000 in 1850 to 50 out of 100,000 by 1950. Improvements in public health were reducing tuberculosis even before the arrival of antibiotics, although the disease's significance was still such that when the Medical Research Council was formed in Britain in 1913 its first project was tuberculosis. Table 2.3 summarizes the timeline of important dates in the detection, prevalence and treatment of tuberculosis during the medieval period.

Table 2.3: Timeline of important dates worldwide in the detection, prevalence and treatment of tuberculosis during medieval period

11th century	Presence of tuberculosis was detected from the mummies of pre-Colombian period in Peru confirming the affliction of people with mycobacterium disease even before the colonization by the Europeans.
1546	Fracastorio suggested that a living contagion was involved in the tuberculosis. Not much was done until the 17th century. Girolamo Tracastoro wrote the book *De Morbis Contagiosis* describing the contagious nature of tuberculosis. He mentioned that bed sheets and clothing of patients could contain contagious particles.
17th century	Postmortem studies showed the importance of the small nodule or 'tubercle' with its tendency to break down into cheesy pus and to ulcerate.
Mid 17th century	One in five deaths in London (according to Bills of Mortality) were due to TB. It even took the form of an epidemic in Britain, major cities of USA and Europe and was known as "White Plague".
1679	Franciscus de la Boe commonly known as Sylvius wrote the *Opera Medica*. This was the first attempt to identify actual tubercles as a consistent and characteristic change in the lungs and other areas of consumptive patients. He also described their progression to abscesses and cavities. Soon thereafter other Italian works began detailing the pathology of the disease and its infectious nature and introduced the need for disinfection of patients, surgical tools, and their belongings.
1699	Earliest reference to the infectious nature of TB in Italian Medical Literature. Anedict issued by the Republic of Lucca stated that "Henceforth, human health should no longer be endangered by objects remaining after the death of a consumptive. The names of the deceased should be reported to the authorities and measures undertaken to disinfections".
1702	Manget described the pathological features of miliary tuberculosis.

Contd...

Table 2.3: Timeline of important dates worldwide in the detection, prevalence and treatment of tuberculosis during medieval period (*Contd...*)

1720	A new theory of consumption was proposed by English Physician Benjamin Marten. According to this TB could be caused by "wonderfully minute living creatures" which, once, they had gained a foothold in the body, could generate the lesions and symptoms of the disease. According to him "It may be therefore very likely that by an habitual lying in the same bed with a consumptive patient, constantly eating and drinking with him, or by very frequently conversing so nearly as to draw in parts of the breath he emits from the lungs, a consumption may be caught by a sound person. I imagine that slightly conversing with consumptive patients is seldom or never sufficient to catch the disease".
1761	Austrian Leopold Avensbrugger wrote a book on tuberculosis wherein the clinical symptoms and different pathologies of the disease were given.
1782	Graumann provided the conclusive proof that syphilis and tuberculosis were not the same disease. Consequently the ban on the use of animals infected with tuberculosis for food was lifted in Prussia (August 1785) and Austria (July 1788).
Beginning 19th century	The estimated annual worldwide TB deaths was 7 million and incidence of pulmonary TB was 50 million. London and New York were two of the worst affected cities. This led to the fear that by the end of the 19th century European civilisation might be destroyed. Shift in the belief about the pathological conditions of tuberculosis occurred. Earlier belief that different conditions represented several diseases were shown to be phases or forms of a single entity.
1810	Transmission of tuberculosis from cattle to humans through infected meat and milk was presented by a London physician, Carmichael.
1848	Brompton hospital for 'consumption' was founded in London.

Contd...

Table 2.3: Timeline of important dates worldwide in the detection, prevalence and treatment of tuberculosis during medieval period (*Contd...*)

1850	Start of Sanatorium system in France In addition to helping treat the ill, it helped in isolating the diseased from the healthy population.
1854	Submission of a doctoral dissertation titled "Tuberculosis is a Curable Disease by Hermann Brehmer a Silesian botany student suffering from TB after being cured by changing his lifestyle and spending time on the advice of his doctor, in the Himalayas. He established the first sanatorium in Gorbersdorf where, in the midst of fir trees and with good nutrition, patients were exposed on their balconies to continuous fresh air. This set up later became the blueprint for establishment of subsequent sanatoria.
1859	Establishment of a sanatorium in Germany thus starting the phase where fresh air, preventive hygienic measures, sputum disinfection and isolation of the patient were gaining favour with health providers. This was strengthened after the discovery made by Koch.
1860	The process of pasteurization was developed in the early 1860s by Louis Pasteur, the French Scientist. It inactivates the bacteria that causes tuberculosis. The introduction of this technique was useful in preventing the transfer of tuberculosis from cows to humans.
1865	French military doctor, Jean-Antoine Villemin demonstrated the specificity and transmissibility of tuberculosis experimentally by transmitting the tuberculosis from humans to cattle to rabbits and postulated that TB was caused by a specific microorganism thus laying to rest the centuries old belief that consumption arose spontaneously in each affected organisms.
1882	Robert Koch, using staining technique, discovered that TB was caused by a bacteria and thus gave the final proof to what JA Villemin postulated in 1865. Koch induced the disease in animals through infecting them with the tubercle bacillus. This became the beginning of the war against humanity's deadliest disease.

Contd...

	Establishment of Sanatorium in US by Dr. Edward Livingston. This was the beginning of a public health movement featuring community participation, emphasis on healthy lifestyle (exercise and nutrition), and ordinances to improve sanitation and slum housing. Voluntary organizations to combat TB were also formed during the sanatorium era. This was a great social movement with both public sector and private sector commitment for halting tuberculosis with good results.
	Direct intervention against TB began with pasteurization of milk and introduction of BCG.
	Active therapy began with the introduction of the artificial pneumothorax and surgical methods to reduce lung volume.
1885	An Italian bacteriologist named Cantani invented a method under which tuberculosis patients inhaled nonpathogenic bacteria to reduce the levels of tuberculoid bacilli in the sputum.
1887	Opening of first specialized dispensary for tuberculosis in Edinburgh by Robert Philip.
1888	The usage of gram-negative bacteria in conjunction with gram-negative bacteria could inhibit the growth of *Mycobacterium tuberculosis*.
1894	C. Forlanini published his first series on artificial pneumothorax. In 1890 he found that collapsing the lungs had positive effect on recovery from tuberculosis. Thereafter doctors began to reduce lung volume to treat tuberculosis.
1895	Discovery of X-ray by Wilhelm Konrad von Rontgen which helped in reviewing the severity and monitoring the progress of the patient's disease. The X-rays were permanent ways to view and record the state of the patient's lung and allowed doctors to see infected areas as well as healing areas.

2.5 MODERN HISTORY OF TUBERCULOSIS (20th century and Later)

Early Treatments

Early Treatment: Physicians have realized that tuberculosis was contagious for centuries. However, it was not until recently, within the last 200 years, that effective treatment methods have been available. Physicians used blood letting or would seek an audience with the king in the hopes of divine healing.

Pneumothorax Treatments

To treat tuberculosis, a lung collapse therapy was developed by an Italian physician Forlanini in 1890. These were of two types. One, the *artificial pneumothorax* included the compression of the diseased lung. The pleural cavities were filled with gas or filtered air. This was repeated daily, with a gradual decrease of treatments. The treatments would be continued sporadically for up to two to four years after the initial treatment. On the other hand, *bilateral pneumothorax* included the compression of both lungs. Only parts of the lungs were collapsed so that patients could still live relatively accurate, normal lives. Two, *thoracoplasty*—This method was more extreme than the previous two. Ribs from one side of the thorax were removed in order to collapse the infected portion of the lung permanently.

Artificial pneumothorax and other forms of lung-collapse therapy were widely used particularly from 1920 onwards when radiographical diagnosis and control became practical and accurate. Much greater emphasis was laid upon the infectious nature of the disease, and upon preventing it by reducing contagion and by insistence on examination of the family contacts. The patients, however, suffered from shortness of breath caused by the decreased lung space. This technique over the years proved to be of little use and was discontinued after 1946 when antibiotics were discovered.

Gold and Other Salts Therapy

During 1925 to 1935, gold therapy had taken the tuberculosis treatment by storm but was soon discarded thereafter. This type of treatment was first introduced in 1925 by Holger Mollgaard in Copenhagen. He developed the compound sanocrysin, a double thiosulphate of gold and sodium. He tested the compound on animals and deemed it safe to use on humans. However, despite claims to the contrary by physicians

Secher and Faber, it was wholly toxic. Danish and British physicians began using smaller doses to combat tuberculosis. Despite smaller doses, it still remained toxic. A test trial was completed in America and proved the toxic effects of gold therapy in 1934. Within a year, most of Europe had ceased to use gold therapy.

From the time of opening of sanatora until the 1940s some of these treatments included the use of iron salts, sodium chloride, calcium chloride, chlorine gas, and iodine. For a long time copper and gold salts were used in the treatment of TB although they proved to have little or no value in the treatment and they also caused injuries to other parts of the body and the skin. Gold salt and sunlight became more widely used after Koch's findings that these two agents inhibited the growth of tubercle bacilli. In light of these findings, light therapy and ultraviolet rays were also used, but they also caused sunburn. It was believed that patients who developed the most pigmentation of the skin from heliotherapy recovered more satisfactorily from extrapulmonary forms of tuberculosis. As time went on and little or no progress was made in finding a cure, efforts were made to develop safer and acceptable methods of treating TB.

Since these treatments could not tackle the infectious nature of the disease, a general reaction against these medications began gaining momentum. With the exception of cod liver oil, Calcium preparation and other items which were useful in relieving symptomatic problems remained in use.

Safer and Acceptable Methods

Environmental Control

During 1935–45, consistent with the economic situation of the countries, health concerns began recognizing the role of environmental factors (poverty, deficient diet, and poor housing) in the incidence and spread of tuberculosis. This led to the development of official schemes of social assistance to tuberculosis patients. Authorities began promoting the widespread use of tuberculin skin tests for diagnosis of infection in cattle and man and on the introduction of mass radiography for diagnosis of unsuspected cases.

Sanatoria

For the treatment and isolation of tuberculosis patients, many sanatoria were established in the 20th century. Initially, there were very few spaces available and they were only open to the elite. By 1950, there were hundreds of thousands of beds available across the United States alone. They were often well maintained and provided rest, fresh air, good food, and a "great mindset" for the patients. With the invention of streptomycin and isoniazid in the 1940s, many of the sanatoria were closed. They were converted to hospitals, religious facilities, and convalescent homes. Several sanatoria had attained negative reputations and were claimed to be haunted and were considered full of "germs". These institutions remained empty for many years following the closure of the sanitorium.

In the early 20th century, the most common age group affected by TB was the elderly. Because TB commonly re-infects the patient, tuberculosis can continually reoccur throughout the patient's life. The widespread use of sanitoria and hospitals to isolate those infected was used to prevent the future generations from contracting the disease. The isolation of the infected people prevented the spread and by 1973 the mortality rate for TB had been dramatically reduced.

Immunization Activities

The first genuine success in immunizing against tuberculosis developed from attenuated bovine strain tuberculosis by Albert Calmette and Camille Guerin in 1906 was BCG (Bacillus of Calmette and Guerin). The duo French bacteriologist used specific culture media to lower the virulence of the bovine TB bacterium. This created the basis for the BCG vaccine which, though relatively ineffective, is still in widespread use today. It was first used on humans on July 18, 1921 in France. National arrogance prevented its widespread use in countries such as the USA, Great Britain, and Germany until after World War II.

BCG Vaccination had been introduced in France and Scandinavia following a survey of 50,000 children which showed an 80% reduction in infection rate. Britain adopted a vaccination programme in the 1950's, America however did not—as their research showed contrary conclusions.

As the public became better educated in the workings of the disease, and the governments took steps to improve housing and poverty, the number of TB cases began dropping, though slowly. It had taken almost three thousand years to understand the full nature of tuberculosis, but the goal of real cure could become visible only when the antibiotics became more sophisticated.

Use of Chemotherapy

Between 1945 and 1960 a remarkable development was made and more patients were cured using the new antibiotics. Now with the disease under control less and less beds were needed. During the 1960s many sanatoria started to close. By the middle of the 1960's there were only a few beds available for patients suffering from TB.

The chemotherapy of infectious diseases, using sulfonamide and penicillin, had been in practice for several years. Unfortunately these were ineffective against *Mycobacterium tuberculosis*. A brief yet useful insight in the treatment of tuberculosis came during the early years of the Second World War. Selman A. Waksman, who had been systematically screening soil bacteria and fungi since 1914, discovered in 1939 the marked inhibitory effect of certain fungi, especially actinomycetes, on bacterial growth. In 1940, he and his team at Rutgers University in New Jersey were able to isolate an effective anti-TB antibiotic, actinomycin; however, this proved to be too toxic for use in humans or animals.

In the USA in 1942, Drs. Feldman and Hinshaw reported the first drug trial (Promin) in the treatment of TB. Unfortunately this trial was unsuccessful due to significant side effects. In January 1944 Drs. Schatz, Bugie and Waksman announced the discovery of a drug called 'Streptomycin' and 'Patricia', a 21 year old woman was the first patient to be successfully treated with the drug.

Success towards treating TB using antibiotics came in 1943. In test animals, it was observed that streptomycin, purified from Streptomyces griseus, led to maximal inhibition of *M. tuberculosis* with relatively low toxicity. On November 20, 1944, the antibiotic was administered for the first time to a critically ill TB patient. The effect was almost immediately impressive. His advanced disease was visibly arrested, the bacteria disappeared from his sputum, and he made a rapid recovery. However, the new drug had side effects – especially on the inner ear – but the fact remained that, *M. tuberculosis* was no longer a bacteriological exception. It was the beginning of a possibility for treating the disease.

The following years saw a rapid succession of anti-TB drugs. These proved useful because with streptomycin as the only medicine available, resistant mutants of tuberculosis bacteria began to appear within a few months of its use. However, it was soon demonstrated that this problem of drug resistance could be overcome with the combination of two or three drugs.

In 1946, a paper was published by Dr. Lehmann concerning the discovery of Para-Amino-Salicylic (PAS) in the treatment of TB and in 1952 at Seaview Hospital, New York, a new wonderdrug called 'Isoniazid' was used to treat TB patients by Drs. Robizek and Selikoff.

In 1960, Dr John Crofton a TB expert at the University of Edinburgh proposed that a combination of drugs, Streptomycin, PAS and Isoniazid made TB completely curable. His proposals to conquer the disease included the pasteurization of milk, tuberculin testing of cattle, BCG vaccinations of whole populations, mass radiography for the early detection of disease, triple therapy for every infected patient, isolation of the infectious and reduction in household overcrowding.

Drug-resistant Tuberculosis

During 1961–1968, a survey in the USA examined drugs susceptibility among TB hospitalized patients. It found that 3.5% patients showed resistance to at least one drug. Subsequently, the USA reported the first outbreak of drug resistant TB in 1970. From then until 1990 the USA experienced a few outbreaks involving small numbers of Isoniazid-resistant and multidrug resistant TB.

Multidrug resistant TB was also reported during 1990–92, by the Center for Disease Control (CDC) in Atlanta USA, which investigated outbreaks of such TB in eight hospitals in Florida, New York and New Jersey. One such case was also reported in the NY State Correctional System. These outbreaks involved large numbers of cases. TB was found to be transmitted not only from patient to patient, but also from patient to health care worker. Also 80% of cases were HIV positive. The first report of MDR-TB outbreak at a London hospital HIV Unit occurred in August 1995—and the second in June 1996.

The prospect of new, faster TB drugs is gaining momentum. Dr Jack Chow, Assistant Director-General of the WHO HIV/AIDS, TB and Malaria cluster and Dr. Mario Raviglione, Director of Stop TB, threw their support behind this critical goal at a meeting of the stakeholders of the Global Alliance for TB Drug Development on 30 October 2003 in Paris. Dr. Chow applauded the stakeholders for embracing a key task that others "would rather walk away from". He added: "The development of new TB drugs will have a profound impact on the way we fight the greatest joint threat now facing us—the combined TB-HIV epidemic".

Directly Observed Therapy System

According to WHO, the recommended way to cure tuberculosis is by means of directly observed therapy (DOT). The DOT system cures more than 95% of individuals with TB, even in the poorest countries; DOT prevents new infections from appearing and it works to help prevent the development of multidrug-resistant TB (MDR-TB). The World Bank identified DOT as one of the most cost effective of all health interventions.

The Recent TB Epidemic

The registered number of new cases of TB worldwide roughly correlates with economic conditions: the highest incidences are seen in those countries of Africa, Asia and Latin America with the lowest gross national products. The World Health Organization estimates that eight million people get TB every year, of whom 95% live in developing countries.

In industrialized countries, the steady drop in TB incidence began to level off in the mid 1980s and then stagnated or even began to increase. Much of this rise can be at least partially attributed to a high rate of immigration from countries with a high incidence of TB.

The rising TB trend is largely influenced by HIV infection. Chances are that only one out of ten immunocompetent people infected with *M. tuberculosis* will fall sick in their lifetimes, but among those with HIV, one in ten per year will develop active TB, while one in two or three tuberculin test positive AIDS patients will develop active TB. In many industrialized countries this is a tragedy for the patients involved, but these cases make up only a small minority of TB cases. In developing countries, the impact of HIV infection on the TB situation, especially in the 20–35 year age group, is of great and increasing concern.

A final factor contributing to the resurgence of TB is the emergence of multidrug resistance. Drug resistance in TB occurs as a result of tubercle bacillus mutations. These mutations are not dependent upon the presence of the drug. Exposed to a single effective anti-TB medication, the predominant bacilli, sensitive to that drug, are killed; the few drug resistant mutants, likely to be present if the bacterial population is large, will, multiply freely. Since it is very unlikely that a single bacillus will spontaneously mutate to resistance to more than one drug, giving multiple effective drugs simultaneously will inhibit the multiplication of these resistant mutants. This is why it is absolutely essential to treat TB patients with the recommended four drug regimen of isoniazid, rifampin, pyrazinamide, and ethambutol or streptomycin.

While wealthy industrialized countries with good public health care systems can be expected to keep TB under control, in much of the developing world a catastrophe awaits. It is crucially important that support be given to research efforts devoted to developing an effective TB vaccine, shortening the amount of time required to ascertain drug sensitivities, improving the diagnosis of TB, and creating new, highly effective anti-TB medications. Without support for such efforts, we run the risk of losing the battle against TB. Table 2.4 presents the timeline of important dates in the detection and treatment of TB-worldwide in modern period.

Table 2.4: Timeline of important dates in the detection and treatment of TB-Worldwide in modern period

1911	Report from British Royal Commission identified three common types of tubercle bacillus, namely, 'human', 'bovine', and 'avian', and that the bovine type also caused disease in man.
1912	Start of National Tuberculosis Scheme in Britain. Thereafter control legislation and official schemes of similar kind were introduced in many countries.
1920	During the early 19th century to the early 20th century, pathogenesis of tuberculosis was being studied. Doctors considered one of the main causes of TB to be stress. A treatise by Assmann during the 1920s cultivated the theory of reinfection, which is earning acceptance among doctors today.
1931	Discovery of BCG (Bacillus Calmett – Guerin) by Drs. Colmetter and Guerin of France.
1938/39	Start of chemotherapy when first success was noted with the synthetic sulphonamide drug sulphanilamide in experimental tuberculosis (1938) and better results obtained by N. Rist with the related sulphone compounds, which, unfortunately, were not reproduced in human tuberculosis.
1940	Selman Waksman cultivated the antibiotics actinomycin and streptothricin but these were highly toxic and could not be administered to patients. The culture used were Actinomycetes, Aspergillus, and Mycotorula.
1942	First drug trial in the treatment of TB was reported by Drs. Fieldman and Hinshaw of USA. Unfortunately, due to significant side effects, the trial was declared unsuccessful.
1943	Streptomycin was purified from Streptomyces griseus to treat TB. Selman A. Waksman developed the antibiotic.
1944	Discovery of a drug called 'Streptomycin' for treatment of TB was announced by Drs. Schatz, Bugie and Waksman. Patricia, a 21 year old woman was the first patient to be successfully treated with the drug which was administered on November 20. The progression of the disease was halted, the bacteria were later absent from the sputum, and the patient was fully healed.

Contd...

Table 2.4: Timeline of important dates in the detection and treatment of TB-Worldwide in modern period (*Contd...*)

1946	Discovery of Para-Amino – Salicylic (PAS) for treatment of TB by Dr. Lahmann. This drug, found to be moderately effective, is still in wide use.
1947	*Mycobacterium tuberculosis* showed, for the first time, resistance to streptomycin.
1948	Combination of streptomycin and PAS is shown to be effective against tuberculosis.
1949	The drug p-aminosalicylic acid is created.
1950	Discovery of the drug thiacetazone.
1951	A new drug, Isoniazid (INH) is created. This drug in combination with PAS was demonstrated to be more effective than the combination of streptomycin and PAS.
1952	First use of "Isoniazid" for treatment of TB by Drs. Robinzek and Selikoff at Seaview Hospital in New York.
1950–60	Beginning of the revolution in the treatment of tuberculosis brought about mainly by chemotherapy. This brought the decline and eventual disappearance of long stay in sanitoria or stay at other places. Also, it brought the end to collapse-therapy procedures in most countries.
1954	The drug pyrazinamide is created.
	Cycloserine is produced.
1960	Declaration of 'all out war' to conquer TB by Dr. John Crofton a TB expert at the University of Edinburgh who declared that TB was curable by combining the drugs "Streptomycm", PAS and Isoniazid.
1962	Ethambutol is created.
1963	Discovery of the drug Rifampicin for treatment of tuberculosis.
1970	Report of first out break of drug resistant TB in USA.
1985–1993	Report on resurgence of tuberculosis in United States when TB cases began to increase steadily and dramatically.
1995–96	Report of MDR -TB outbreak at a London hospital HIV Unit.

2.6 HISTORICAL DEVELOPMENTS OF TUBERCULOSIS IN INDIA

India's fight against TB is nearly a century old. It began as a sanatorium-based activity founded by voluntary organizations, which soon enlarged its scope to a community-based public health programme, aided by the proactive role of the government. It evolved from purely preventive and educative activities to include curative services[1].

The developments related to management and control of TB in India lagged international efforts by about more than a century. Early measures at best could be classified as preventive and protective. Initially these were aimed at regaining apparent healthy condition and extending longevity, if possible. The scientific management, after the detection of the infectious nature of the disease, largely depended on preventive methods through isolation of TB patients and was started almost about a century ago. Introduction of curative work leading to control and/or eradication of the disease was achieved much later. However, recognition of the TB problem in India could come only as late as 1912 after a resolution passed at All India Sanitary Conference held in Madras (now Chennai) in 1912. The quantitative picture of the disease emerged only after the introduction of tuberculin testing much later. The Bhore committee in its report issued in 1946 estimated that about 2.5 million patients in India at that time required treatment where only 6,000 beds were available.

The historical developments related to tuberculosis in India may, for convenience, be segmented into two broad periods: one, as pre-chemotherapy period and two, the post-chemotherapy period. These may further be sub-divided depending upon our specific interest. The following sub-groups provide a better idea of the developments: opening of sanatorium; role of BCG; establishment of specific institutions; data gathering; post-chemotherapy period (development of infrastructure,

[1]SP Agarwal, Sophia Vijay, P. Kumar, LS Chauhan: The History of Tuberculosis Control in India: Glimpses through Decades, in Tuberculosis Control in India, (ed.), SP Agarwal and LS Chauhan, Directorate General of Health Services, Ministry of Health and Family Welfare, Government of India.

policies and programmes). For convenience of readers, a timeline of important developments in the management (prevention, control, etc.) of tuberculosis in India is presented in Table 2.5.

2.6.1 Establishment of Sanatoriums

As stated earlier, since there was no breakthrough in the treatment of TB for a long time in the world as a whole, Indian infrastructure had to provide facilities consistent with the conditions prevailing in the world at the time, although with substantial time lag. As the only available mode of treatment was isolation, providing good food and ventilation in a sanatorium, a number of such facilities were developed. This was in line with the practice in Europe during pre-chemotherapeutic era. The first open air sanatorium for treatment and isolation of TB patients in India was founded in 1906 in Tiluania, near Ajmer (Rajasthan). A couple of years later, another one, following the design of the earlier one, opened in Almora (Uttarakhand) in 1908. The first non-missionary sanatorium was built near Shimla in 1909. Based on the work done by Dr. Louis Hart beginning 1908, the United Mission Tuberculosis Sanatorium (UMTS) was built in 1912 at Madanapalle, south India.

In the absence of any effective drug or combination of drugs against TB till middle of the 20th century, the main line of treatment continued to be providing good food, extending open air and dry climate to the patients. Till the advent of adequate chemotherapy, treatment took a second place to diagnosis and prognosis. Under the prevailing circumstances and soon after its formation in 1939, the Tuberculosis Association of India (TAI) recommended the Organized Home Treatment Scheme for management of tuberculosis. This was claimed to be the best compromise at that time.

2.6.2 Role of BCG

BCG (Bacillus Calmette Guerin) Campaign in India

BCG vaccine was used extensively in many of the European countries beginning in the 1920s and was the most important

Table 2.5: Timeline in the control of tuberculosis in India

1906	Founding of the first open air sanatorium for treatment and isolation of TB patients in Tiluania, near Ajmer, (Rajasthan)
1908	Establishment of TB Sanatorium, on the line of that at Tiluania, in Almora, (Uttarakhand).
1909	Establishment of first non-missionary sanatorium near Shimla, (Himachal Pradesh).
1912	Establishment of United Mission Tuberculosis Sanatorium at Madanapalle, South India. This was based on the work done by Dr. Louis Hart in 1908.
	Recognition of the TB problem in India through a resolution passed in the All India Sanitary Conference, held at Madras (now Chennai).
1917	Opening of first TB dispensary in Bombay (now Mumbai) followed by another in Madras (now Chennai).
1929	India became member of the International Union against Tuberculosis (IUAT). This was done on the basis of recommendation by DR Lankaster to government that it (the government) should work closely with non-governmental organizations to control TB.
	Formation of Bengal TB Association.
	Organisation of King George V Thanksgiving (anti TB) Fund for control of the disease in the country. The fund was used through the Indian Red Cross Society for preventive and educational activities, establishment of clinics, training of health visitors and preparation of health education material.
1937	Issue of a public appeal for anti-TB funds on behalf of the Government by Her Excellency Lady Linlithgow. Five percent of the money collected was retained at the centre and the balance was distributed to the provinces and states.
1939	Formation of TB Association of India (TAI) on February 23. This was followed by formation of TB Associations by provinces and states which received money from the fund raised in 1937. TAI used the Anti-TB Funds raised in 1929 and 1937 and recommended the Organized Home Treatment Scheme for TB as the best compromise under the prevailing circumstances.

Contd...

Table 2.5: Timeline in the control of tuberculosis in India (*Contd...*)

1946	Publication of Report of Bhore Committee where Organised Home Treatment Scheme was given priority and setting up of a clinic for each district and use of mobile clinics for rural areas was recommended.
1947	Creation of a TB Division in the Directorate General of Health Services (DGHS) in New Delhi with an adviser in TB as its head.
1948	Start of a pilot project at two centres for assessing the use and effectiveness of BCG (Bacillus Calmette Guerin).
	Setting up of a BGG Vaccination Production Centre in Guindy, Madras with support from WHO and UNICEF.
1949	Pilot BCG testing extended to schools in almost all states of India.
1951	Start of a mass BCG campaign in India. Sixty five million children vaccinated, 165 million tuberculin tests administered.
1956	Establishment of Tuberculosis Chemotherapy Center later known as Tuberculosis Research Centre (TRC) in Madras (Chennai) under the auspices of Indian Council of Medical Research (ICMR), Government of Madras, WHO and the British Medical Research Council (BMRC).
1955–58	Under the auspices of the ICMR a large-scale sample survey was conducted in six zones of the country covering both urban and rural populations, to obtain as precise information as possible about the magnitude of the TB problem in the country. The survey revealed high prevalence rate of TB (prevalence of sputum positive pulmonary TB to be about 4 per 1,000 population with 80% being in rural areas).
1959	Establishment of the National TB Institute (NTI) in Bangalore by Government of India with the active cooperation of the WHO. The Institute was to develop a TB control programme which could be operationally feasible, applicable to both rural and urban areas, economically affordable and promised substantial benefits to the community.
1961	Pilot testing of national tuberculosis programme (NTP) in Ananthpur district of Andhra Pradesh. This was to take care of epidemiological, sociological, operational, technical and administrative aspects of the TB control in India.

Contd...

Table 2.5: Timeline in the control of tuberculosis in India (*Contd...*)

1962	Launch of National Tuberculosis Programme (NTP).
1968	Decision by Government of India to assess the efficacy of BCG vaccination by carrying out a clinical trial in Chingleput district of Tamil Nadu. The study revealed that BCG did not offer protection against pulmonary TB. However, despite this finding a decision was taken to continue with BCG vaccination in children as a part of the expanded programme of immunisation (EPI) to provide protection against the serious childhood forms of TB.
1992	Review of the performance of national tuberculosis programme (NTP) by Government of India along with WHO and SIDA which showed that despite technical soundness, NTP suffered from managerial weaknesses, inadequate funding, an over-reliance on X-ray for diagnosis, had frequent interrupted supplies of drugs and low rates of treatment completion.
1992–93	First round of National Family Health Survey (NFHS-1) included a question on the prevalence of TB in the households. Based on the basis of information given by either head or a responsible person in the household, the report gives the prevalence of TB in various states of India.
1993	Launch of revised national TB control programme (RNTCP) based on internationally recommended strategy of directly observed treatment short-course (DOTS) by WHO. This was to rectify the limitations of NTP.
1998-99	NFHS-2 repeats the question on prevalence of TB along with the prevalence of medically treated TB and gives the information at state level.
2000-03	National sample survey to estimate the annual risk of tuberculosis infection (ARTI) conducted by National TB Institute, Bangalore, in collaboration with TB Research Centre, Chennai and the concerned states in four zones of the country. The national ARTI level was estimated as 1.5 percent (2.1 percent urban and 1.3 per cent rural).
2005-06	NFHS-3 repeats the questions on TB in the form used in NFHS-2.
2006	Launch of Second Phase of RNTCP (October).
2007-09	Second round of ARTI survey launched in January 2007 and to be completed by 2009 is to provide new estimates of the measures to assess the prevalence of TB in the country.

vaccine for protection and prevention of tuberculosis. Use of BCG in India started in a pilot project implemented in two centers in 1948. In 1949, it was extended to schools in almost all states of India. Under the aegis of the International Tuberculosis Campaign with considerable experience in BCG work in many countries, it was introduced in India on a small scale in Madanapalle with Dr. Frimodt Moller in the lead. India started a mass BCG Campaign in 1951. A BCG Vaccine Production Center with assistance from WHO and UNICEF was set up in Guindy, Chennai in 1948.

Controlled Clinical Trial for Efficacy of BCG Vaccine

BCG vaccination was the only available protective measure against TB. Different trials had not revealed credible proof of its efficacy. Controversy on the protective effect of BCG lingered as the studies carried out in different countries showed that the protective effect varied between 0 to 80%. Many, including late Sri C Rajagopalachari, even though that its efficacy was not fully proven and strongly advocated against its continued large-scale use. It would be in the interest of the country to undertake a well designed trial to seek clear answers to the major issues confronting it. Therefore, the National Tuberculosis Institute (NTI) had been vigorously planning to conduct a major BCG trial and had even reserved certain areas in the country as vaccination-free zones. It was in touch with the international scientific community, various vaccine production centres and in the field. In January 1964, it initiated intensive discussions with the WHO experts and representatives from United States Public Health Service (USPHS). It was agreed that any trial undertaken was not to interfere with the progress of NTI and National Tuberculosis Programme (NTP); and also since such a trial was expensive and prolonged, it had to be designed with utmost care and efficiency.

Ultimately, the project named Feasibility Study for TB Prevention Trials became part of the Indian Council of Medical Research (ICMR) and moved out of the campus to its own building. In time, its studies showed that the major BCG trial would be best if conducted in Chingleput district of Tamil Nadu than in other areas reserved for the purpose. Field work began and the office was moved to Madras. In spite of shifting of the project camp to Madras, NTI continued to assist the BCG Trial by providing technical guidance and replacement of staff. When Dr. Raj Narain, Epidemiologist of NTI retired, Dr. Baily, TB Specialist of NTI joined as the Director of this study and continued to serve till the first report was published.

The BCG trial was completed as scheduled. After a period of twelve and a half years, it brought out a revolutionary report. It showed that BCG vaccination did not offer significant protection against TB of the lung. Several expert committees appointed both by the authorities in India and by the WHO examined all the procedures followed up in the study and came to the conclusion that the study had been meticulously carried out and vaccine used in the trial were the best available ones. The implications of this study was: Should BCG vaccination be given up in India? Another committee appointed jointly by ICMR and the WHO went into the epidemiological aspects of the causation of TB under Indian conditions. It concluded that though BCG may not protect against TB of lung which occurs mostly in adults, it could provide substantial protection against childhood forms of TB such as tubercular meningitis, miliary TB. The protective effect of BCG against these forms of TB was not studied in Chingleput Trial. In India BCG vaccination policy was revised and it was recommended to be given at an early age preferably before the end of the first year after birth by integrating under Universal Immunization Programme (UIP). BCG vaccination policies in many other countries were also revised as a consequence of the Chingleput study findings.

2.6.3 Institutional Developments

Government Organizations

Dr. Frimodt Moller, the first Medical Superintendent, played a large role in India's fight against TB through the training of TB workers, conducting TB surveys (1939) and introduction of BCG vaccination (1948). In addition, the first TB dispensary was opened in Bombay in 1917, followed by another in Chennai. Soon anti-TB societies were formed in Lucknow and Ajmer.

For India, which included Pakistan and Bangladesh in most of the first half of the twentieth century, the small scale and irregular efforts of NGOs in tackling the issues related to tuberculosis were not adequate. It was essential for the government to take initiative. Despite the consensus reached, the issue of diagnosis, let alone treatment, remained unresolved for a long time. Only by 1925, chest radiology could detect a deep-seated area of TB consolidation and thoracic surgeons began to demand X-rays. The capability of the apparatus to embody the MMR version could be reached only by 1945. In the meantime the Second World War broke out and fighting disease took a back seat.

The Bhore Committee report in 1946 was a land mark event in the management and treatment of tuberculosis. It had estimated that there were about 2.5 million patients in the country who required treatment. It also reported that in 1946 there were only 6000 beds available for the treatment of TB patients. Further, the country was experiencing about one-half million deaths due to TB annually. In order to provide adequate treatment facilities for the treatment of TB this wide gap between the number of patients and hospital beds had to be bridged. With this turn of events and keeping in view the sheer magnitude of the disease, it was felt that the government should be a key player in initiating measures to control the disease. The committee recommended establishment of an organized domiciliary service by setting up of TB clinics in the districts and mobile TB clinics for rural areas. Around the same time, a TB Division in the Directorate General of Health Services (DGHS), was established in New Delhi in 1946, with an Adviser in TB as its head. TB was also given a prominent place in the planning. Since the government was not only concerned with TB but with other diseases and health infrastructure, it constituted a committee under the chairmanship of Sir Joseph Bhore. Its secretary was Rai Bahadur KCKE Raja, who as the Director General of Health Services (DGHS) played a dominant role in the TB field during his tenure.

Research and Development

On the initiative of Dr Benjamin the Tuberculosis Chemotherapy Centre (TCC), now known as Tuberculosis Research Centre (TRC) was established in Chennai in 1956. The Centre was started under the auspices of the Indian Council of Medical Research, Government of Madras at that time, the World Health Organization (WHO) and the British Medical Research Council (BMRC). This Center was to provide information on the mass domiciliary application of chemotherapy in the treatment of pulmonary TB. In this context, the Center carried out an epoch-making study and demonstrated that the time-honoured virtues of sanatorium treatment such as bed rest, well-balanced diet and good accommodation were remarkably unimportant provided adequate chemotherapy was prescribed and taken. The study also showed that there was no evidence that close family contacts of patients treated at home incurred an increased risk of contracting TB. These findings paved the way for considering the appropriateness of treating infectious patients in their own homes and therefore, it was logical to formulate a nationally applicable TB control programme in the country on that line. The finding also brought a revolution in the treatment of TB patients in the world.

The Government of India with the cooperation of the World Health Organization established a National Tuberculosis Institute (NTI) in 1959 at Bangalore (now Bengaluru). The institute, started under the dynamic leadership of Dr. PV Benjamin, was established primarily to formulate a programme for TB control, training of district TB key personnel and orientation training for medical officers and paramedical TB workers. The conditions for the programme were that it should be operationally feasible, applicable to both the rural and urban areas of the entire country, economically affordable and offered substantial benefits to the community.

With available resources, though limited, the National TB Control Programme (NTCP) formulated in 1962 and implemented throughout the country was to create a good infrastructure in most parts of the country. A large number of key personnel of District TB Centres were trained in carrying out NTCP activities. It was also engaged in monitoring the TB control programme and providing feedback from time to time both to the central and state authorities. The Institute has conducted several important studies on different aspects of TB disease: epidemiological, operational, sociological and bacteriological. These findings have been found useful in improving the TB control strategies.

Non-Governmental Organizations

Tuberculosis Association of India

In view of the high prevalence and inadequate facilities available in the country to deal with tuberculosis related problems, Dr. Lankaster recommended that the government should work closely with the non-governmental organizations (NGOs) and support their activities. In response to this suggestion, India became a member of the International Union Against Tuberculosis (IUAT) in 1929. In another related development in 1937, Her Excellency Lady Linlithgow issued a public appeal for anti-TB funds on behalf of the government. As a result, the King Emperor's Anti-Tuberculosis Fund collected nearly a crore of rupees. A token 5% of this money was retained by the center and the balance was distributed to the provinces and states. The 5% of the money retained from the above direct donations along with funds obtained from the King George V Thanksgiving (Anti-TB) Fund was used to establish The TB Association of India (TAI) in February, 1939 as a registered society. The provinces and states which received money also started their TB associations. The Bengal TB Association, however, which started functioning in 1929, maintained dispensaries in Calcutta (now Kolkata) and Howrah. Additional funds were used to strengthen its activities. The membership of TAI included the state affiliates who nominated their representatives to its Annual General Meeting and Central Committee. Dr. C Frimodt Moller and Dr. BK Sikand took a lead in starting the association.

The objectives of TAI include the following:

- Prevention, control and treatment of tuberculosis and relief from the disease.
- Encouragement of and assistance in the establishment throughout India of State Associations having objectives similar in whole or in part to those of the TAI.
- Affiliation or control of and the rendering of assistance to any institution having objectives similar in whole or in part to the objects of the TAI.
- Undertaking of Research and Investigation on subjects concerning tuberculosis and allied chest diseases.
- Undertaking such things as are incidental or conducive to the attainment of the above objectives.

Some of the major activities of the TAI are:

- Providing quality diagnostic and treatment services through the New Delhi TB Centre.
- Complementing/supplementing Revised National Tuberculosis Control Program and Directly Observed Treatment Short Course services of Government of India.
- Carrying out a TB Seal Campaign inaugurated every year on 2nd October by the President of India, the Patron of TAI, to solicit funds for supporting its activities. The Association does not receive any Government funds. This seal has won 'First Prize of TB Seal Designs' by the International Union Against Tuberculosis and Lung Diseases, Paris, for the years 2006 and 2007.
- Holding of national and state level conferences for promoting technical education and updating knowledge of tuberculosis.
- Production of films, flip charts, street plays to boost the IEC activities and publication of relevant literature and research findings.

New Delhi TB Center

The New Delhi Tuberculosis Centre was started in 1940 to serve as a model clinic. This was a joint venture of the Tuberculosis Association of India and Government of India. This centre was planned to try the concept of domiciliary treatment scheme developed by Dr. BK Sikand, the first Director of the Centre and Dr. C. Frimodt Moller. Later in 1951, with the assistance from WHO, UNICEF and Government of India, the clinic was upgraded to become the first TB Training and Demonstration Centre in the country.

The Centre provides teaching and training facilities to the under-graduate students of Maulana Azad Medical College (MAMC), Interns of Lok Nayak Hospital and post Graduate students of Vallabhbhai Patel Chest Institute, Delhi University. It has two modular training programmes: one in tuberculosis for fresh graduates and interns of MAMC, and two in Bio-Statistics for medical post graduate students of Delhi University. To deal with the menace of Multi Drug-resistant TB a specialized clinic was started in the Centre in August, 2002. Its laboratory is renowned for various TB related tests and receives samples from different parts of the country.

The Centre runs a TB Health Visitor course of nine months duration for students from Delhi and various other states of the country. It also imparts training to nursing students from various institutions such as Lok Nayak Hospital, Ram Manohar Lohia Hospital, Sir Ganga Ram Hospital, Lady Harding Health School and Rajkumari Amrit Kaur College of Nursing.

Further, it is actively involved with the implementation of the Revised National TB Control Programme (RNTCP) since January, 1999. It has two DOTS cum Microscopy Centres and two DOTS Centres to carry out the programme. In addition, it is providing modular training to medical officers, senior tuberculosis laboratory supervisors and laboratory technicians.

Further, it is engaged in the dissemination of knowledge about tuberculosis prevention and control among general population through community meetings. It also conducts health education through flip charts and video films. The Centre mobilizes assistance to the poor patients and their families from a number of agencies. Research work and library facilities at the Centre add a very useful dimension to the prevention and control of tuberculosis.

2.6.4 Data Collection

National Sample Surveys Related to Tuberculosis

In 1950, Dr. PV Benjamin reported that tuberculosis infection is so widespread that no part of the country is free from it. The subsequent BCG campaigns revealed similar findings. However, this needed to be checked by scientifically conducted surveys. For a country as large as India, the sample of one area was inadequate. Reliable information on the magnitude and extent of the disease in the various cross sections of the population was required. This was not an easy task. Apart from resources, trained personnel to conduct large – scale surveys was not readily available. A special committee of the ICMR was set up to address the issue of obtaining this information expeditiously and rationally. It decided that a systematic survey on a countrywide basis should be undertaken.

Prevalence of tuberculosis survey: To obtain as precise information as possible about the magnitude of the TB problem in India, a large–scale sample survey was conducted in the country under the auspices of the Indian Council of Medical Research. Dr. PV Benjamin, as a member of the Health Planning Cell in the Planning Commission, was instrumental in initiating this National Sample Survey that extended from 1955 to 1958. The survey included the six zones in which the country was divided for the survey and covered both urban and rural populations. The findings revealed that the problem of TB was uniformly distributed, both in the urban and rural population of the country. The results revealed a high prevalence rate for TB (prevalence of sputum positive pulmonary TB to be about 4 per 1,000 persons with 80% being in rural areas). The X-ray active cases were estimated at 16 per 1000 persons.

Annual risk of tuberculosis infection (ARTI): In view of the importance of ARTI in any programme directed towards tuberculosis control, lack of any reliable data for the entire country and the cost involved in collecting data, the government of India implemented the programme to conduct a nation-wide tuberculosis survey during 2000–03. This was the time when the tuberculosis control activities were being intensified under the RNTCP. The objective of the survey was to estimate the prevalence of infection among children one to nine years of age and to compute average ARTI in each of the four defined zones into which the country was stratified for the purpose of the survey. The survey was conducted independently in each zone (north, south, east and west) following a uniform methodology, with NTI (National TB Institute, Bangalore) as the nodal centre and TRC (TB Research Centre), Chennai, as the collaborating centre with local support from state health authorities. Two different methods were used to estimate the prevalence of tuberculosis infection.

In view of the importance of the estimate of ARTI in TB control programme, India will be conducting the second large–scale country-wide study to ascertain the number of people who fall prey to tuberculosis every year. This next round of ARTI survey to be carried out during 2007–2009, beginning January 2007, is to cover about 300,000 children. This sample size is about 50% larger than that in the first round of the survey. The findings are expected to provide the clearer picture of the effectiveness of the TB control programme implemented through DOTS strategy currently in use. The survey, like the earlier one, will be conducted by the Tuberculosis Research Centre, Chennai and the National Tuberculosis Institute, Banglore. The findings of this survey hopefully will provide truer picture of the prevalence of tuberculosis in India and its various regions compared to that noted in the first ARTI survey.

National family health survey: There is limited experience in collecting large scale morbidity data through population based demographic surveys in India. However, an attempt was made in the First Round of the National Family Health Survey conducted during 1992–93 (NFHS-1), to collect data on five major morbidity conditions including tuberculosis. During the field work of the survey, the household head or other knowledgeable adult in the household reported morbidity condition for each household member. No effort was made to do clinical tests for the disease condition. Since the results relating to prevalence of tuberculosis in particular from the survey were found to be generally plausible, the question on morbidity was retained in the subsequent rounds of the

National Family Health Survey–Second Round conducted during 1998–99 (NFHS-2) and Third Round conducted during 2006–06 (NFHS-3). To improve the understanding of the extent of prevalence of tuberculosis in the population in the country and its various regions, NHFS-2 and NFHS-3 expanded the question on tuberculosis to cover the prevalence of medically treated TB along with that reported as in NFHS-1. NFHS-3 conducted during 2005–06 provides data on prevalence of TB in India, comparable to that given by NFHS-2. In addition this round also provides information on knowledge and attitude towards TB. The details from this source are reviewed in chapter three while analysing the status of TB in India.

2.6.5 Period of Conventional Chemotherapy

The very notion that there could be effective drugs against the tubercle bacilli was so revolutionary that researchers began to experiment on the effective dosages and combinations of drugs to be used. The development of anti-TB drugs was chequered and sporadic over a period of two decades starting from 1940s. Streptomycin (SM) and Para-Amino Salicylic Acid (PAS) were first introduced in 40s followed by Thioacetazone and Isonicotinic Acid Hydrazide (INH) in 50s. The issue of affordability was also considered. In the 1949, Annual TB Workers Conference, several papers were presented on the effects of PAS and SM on the patients and on the distribution of SM in India. In 1952, Drs. Robitzek and Selikoff revealed that INH is a miracle drug against TB and it continues as such till date. This gave a global impetus for treatment and control of TB. In 1951, these drugs were tried out on smaller scale in a limited number of patients in India by Dr. Sikand from New Delhi TB Centre, Dr. Sen from Calcutta in 1952, Dr. Frimodt Moller from Madanapalle in 1953, and Dr. Sikand and Dr. Pamra from Delhi in 1956.

In 1953, Frimodt Moller reported remarkable results with the regimen SM and INH, single and combined, in the treatment of pulmonary TB in Indian patients. In 1956, Drs. Sikand and Pamra presented a paper on the "effect of SM, PAS and INH in 703 cases of pulmonary TB, diagnosed and treated during

1951–53". They found that the results of domiciliary treatment were encouraging enough to warrant a shift of emphasis from hospitals and sanatoria to clinics without waiting for any further trials.

These studies would, in time, revolutionize the management of TB all over the world. However, it soon became apparent that the tubercle bacilli could not be destroyed easily even with drugs. They had powerful survival techniques, besides developing resistance to drugs. Trials indicated that the newly available drugs, when used singly, were effective only for short periods. To be effective, conventional treatment had to be continued for at least 12–18 months. This brought with it several problems. How many patients would continue to take medicines for such a long duration? How to keep track? Further research was, therefore, needed to harness the potential of these newly discovered drugs.

The National Tuberculosis Control Programme (NTP)

The operational research studies conducted by the National TB Institute (NTI) paved the way for enunciation of suitable methods for the large-scale application of TB control measures. Based on the recommendations it was necessary that the control programme was taken out of the hands of specialists as was the case until that time and integrated into general health services. They also helped orient services towards chest symptomatics in the community who sought relief from their suffering from general health institutions. Thus the National TB Control Programme (NTP) was formulated to take into account factors related to the epidemiological, sociological, operational, technical and administrative aspects of TB control in India. To make the TB control programme more effective, a new meaning was given to it which was backed by scientifically conceived 'felt needs'. An entirely new dimension in community perception and participation was added under the programme. This approach diverted attention away from the TB sanatoria and rehabilitation centers, and directed the same towards the primary need of providing reliable and prompt diagnosis, domiciliary treatment and preventive services for the entire population. The Programme required testing before it could be launched on an all India basis.

An integrated NTP was pilot tested in Ananthpur district of Andhra Pradesh during 1961. Subsequently, it was launched in a phased manner throughout the country to cover 364 districts using five different (R1 to R5) regimen. Monitoring was taken up initially on a regional basis. Later NTI took up the monitoring work for the entire country. From the analysis of monitoring reports and the observations made in a number of studies, it stood out prominently that the compliance with anti-TB treatment for 12 to 18 months was a big problem under field conditions. This was of great concern particularly when researchers had already demonstrated the possibility of bringing down the duration of treatment to as low as 6 to 8 months.

District TB Programme

Based on the findings of the operational studies conducted, a draft recommendation for the District Tuberculosis Programme (DTP) was prepared in 1961, keeping in mind an average Indian district, its population and health facilities available. The national policy as enunciated in the introduction manual of DTP implementing domiciliary treatment comprised:

- Use of a standard drug regimen of 12–18 months duration;
- Treatment free of cost;
- Priority to newly diagnosed patients, over previously treated patients;
- Treatment organization fully decentralized;
- Efficient defaulter system/mostly self-administered regimen;
- Timely follow up; and
- Chemoprophylaxis not recommended as it was impractical on mass basis.

Social sciences were consciously included as hard evidence and peoples voices were placed on par with science, technology and administration. The National Programme was fully integrated with the government health services of the country, thus extending the scope of TB work to be available through its vast reaches.

Anantapur district was chosen to establish the first model district TB centre (DTC). This programme aimed at the integration of TB control schemes with the existing government health services to reduce the TB problem in the community as economically as possible. In the DTC, the X-ray examination facilities were provided on three days in a week and sputum examination daily.

Shortly after establishing the Anantapur DTC it became evident that case finding could be done at any place without difficulty but the major problem was that of keeping the patients on continuous treatment. Considerable time and effort was devoted to solve the problem of default. Only 66% of the TB patients were taking drugs regularly with a defaulter rate varying from 20% to 54%, with an overall average at 34%.

The Anantapur DTC became operational quickly and functioned well because, in addition to the state government's component, NTI staff also worked. By October 1961, NTI trainers and trainees withdrew. From then on, there was a decline in the services of this DTP. The Anantapur programme suffered from not being recognized by the Andhra State government as essentially their responsibility.

It was not possible to measure disease burden accurately through monitoring. However, it was considered important to evaluate the performance of the units of the DTPs in an ongoing manner and take corrective action simultaneously. This was expected to improve the programme efficiency on a regular basis. Till 1978 monitoring of the programme was done by northern and southern regional centers and from then by NTI only.

The Evaluation of the NTP

The National Tuberculosis Control Programme (NTP) had by 1978 covered 390 (81% of the total districts) in the country. It was using the conventional treatment regimens of 12–18 months which was developed through chemotherapy trials. Initially monitoring of the programme was done on a regional basis. Later, it was taken up by the NTI for the entire country. Monitoring reports and observational studies conducted in field conditions relating to the programme revealed that the treatment compliance in the programme was not up to the desired level.

To improve the compliance rate a new regimen was introduced. It depended upon the availability of Rifampicin, and the reintroduction of Pyrazinamide. The combination was found to bring desired results by reducing the duration of treatment in clinical trials. It was thus possible to reduce the duration of treatment under this six-month short-course chemotherapy (SCC) regimen from twelve to six months. With the introduction of SCC regimens, a new era had started in the fight against TB. However, before a large scale adoption the new regimen required assessment of its feasibility. Thus in 1983, TRC, Chennai, conducted a pilot test in 18 districts of the country to assess the feasibility of SCC implementation on a larger scale. Successful SCC field trials by TRC and NTI paved the way for Government of India to agree for the introduction of SCC in 1986 on a wider scale in the country and subsequently 252 districts were covered.

The costly intervention alone, however, could not improve the treatment compliance which increased only marginally. Despite the NTP being in existence since 1962, no appreciable change in the epidemiological situation of TB in the country had been observed. The HIV-AIDS epidemic and the spread of multidrug resistance TB were threatening to further worsen the situation. To find a solution to the nagging issue of improving the treatment compliance a number of agencies were involved in its evaluation aimed at review of the TB situation and the performance of NTP. Between 1975 and 1992, three independent agencies carried out these studies. These are: the ICMR in 1975; the Institute of Communication, Operations Research and Community Involvement (ICORCI) in 1988; and Government of India with assistance from WHO and the Swedish International Development Agency (SIDA) in 1992. These evaluations noted the wide gap between expected and actual achievements of the programme. Specifically the findings revealed that the NTP, though technically sound, suffered from managerial weaknesses, inadequate funding, an over-reliance on X-ray for diagnosis, frequent interruption in supply of drugs, non-standard treatment regimens, lack of systematic information on treatment outcomes and low rates of treatment completion. To rectify these lacunae, the Government decided to give a new thrust to TB control activities by revitalizing the NTP, with assistance from international agencies, in 1993. To overcome these difficulties, the Revised National Tuberculosis Control Programme (RNTCP) was designed.

The NTI had believed in assessment and evaluation as an ongoing process. It welcomed the idea of periodic assessment, especially from experts, on scientific lines as they were vital to the growth and improvement in the programme.

Era of Short Course Chemotherapy

Chemotherapy of TB underwent revolutionary changes in the seventies owing to the availability of two well-tolerated and highly effective drugs–rifampicin and pyrazinamide. These drugs allowed short course chemotherapy (SCC) and made it possible to simplify treatment and reduce its duration. Discovery of rifampicin in 1967 is considered as one of the greatest achievements in the history of development of anti-TB drugs. After its discovery no new drug has been found. Use of SCC made RNTCP a success as given below.

Formulation of the RNTCP

Based on the recommendations and taking cognizance of concerns expressed by the Central Health Council, the Government of India, with assistance from World Bank, took steps in 1993 to implement the Revised National TB Control Programme (RNTCP) in selected areas. The new format incorporated the strengths and accom-plishments of the National Tuberculosis Programme (NTP), which had created an extensive infrastructure for tuberculosis control in the country, with a network of 446 District TB Centres, 330 TB Clinics and more than 47,600 TB beds. The NTP also raised awareness of TB and TB treatment facilities, and had succeeded in placing more than 13 lakh patients on treatment on a yearly basis. The revised programme adopted the internationally recommended directly observed treatment short-course

(DOTS) strategy which was hailed as the most systematic and cost-effective approach to revitalize the TB control programme in the country.

The infrastructure developed under NTP was strengthened and decentralized for implementation of RNTCP. The supervision and managerial responsibilities were also decentralized and new posts were created. To achieve this, a sub-district-level supervisory team (known as the TB Unit) was created. This team comprised of a treatment supervisor (Senior Treatment Supervisor, STS) and a laboratory supervisor (Senior TB Laboratory Supervisor, STLS). In addition, a medical officer from the general health system was designated to serve as Medical Officer—TB Control at sub-district level who had to shoulder TB control duties in addition to other duties. These 3 individuals constituted the management unit responsible for overseeing operations covering approximately 5 lakh persons and 5 designated microscopy centers. The team was made mobile with the help of a vehicle/POL inputs. Each microscopy centre was equipped with a state-of-the art binocular microscope, good quality reagents and new recording and reporting proformae. To ensure the quality, the programme implemented intensive modular training, supervision, and cross-checking of the work of the laboratory technicians.

RNTCP implementation began in October 1993 and covered a population of 2.35 million spread over 5 sites in different states (Delhi, Kerala, West Bengal, Maharashtra, and Gujarat). It was expanded to cover a population of 13.85 million in 1995 and 16 million in 1996. Subsequently the project was implemented in a phased manner to ensure that quality of services was maintained. As shown below by March 2006 the entire country was under the programme.

Year	1998	1999	2000	2001	2002	2003	2004	2005	2006
Population Covered*	18	130	287	450	530	775	947	1080	1114

*Cumulative, in millions

Achievements of RNTCP

- Entire country now has access to DOTS. In terms of treatment of patients, RNTCP is the largest and the fastest expanding programme in the world. Quality of services has been maintained during this rapid expansion.
- In 1999, the Indian expansion of RNTCP accounted for 1/3 and in 2000 and 2001 for over 1/2 of the global increase in DOTS coverage. In 2004 alone, more than 1 million TB patients were initiated on treatment.
- Sound training materials were developed for all categories of staff. The training materials are modular in content to ensure standard quality training and to avoid possible subjectivity and bias of the trainers.
- Diagnostic facilities in more than 11,000 laboratories throughout the country have been established.
- Treatment success rates have tripled from 25% to 86%. TB death rates have been cut 7-fold from 29% to 4%.
- Since its inception, the Programme has initiated over 5.4 million patients on treatment, thus saving nearly one million additional lives.
- During the year 2005, a number of new initiatives listed below were taken:
  - Initiation of a 'referral for treatment' mechanism in 12 districts with large medical colleges, aiming at developing seamless RNTCP service between medical colleges and general health services.
  - Finalization of external quality assessment (EQA) protocol and revised RNTCP EQA guidelines.
  - Finalization of drug resistant surveillance (DRS) protocol.
  - DOTS Plus guidelines developed for starting treatment of MDR TB cases.
  - Patient-wise boxes (PWBs) for paediatric patients were developed. This was the unique global achievement for RNTCP, as no other DOTS programme in the world had such PWBs for the treatment of children with tuberculosis.
  - Training modules on TB-HIV issues were developed jointly with the National AIDS Control Programme.

- HIV surveillance in TB patients in four districts.
- Disease prevalence and mortality surveys initiated.
- State specific Annual Risk of TB Infection (ARTI) surveys started.

Second Phase of RNTCP

In the first phase of RNTCP (1998–2005), the programme's focus was on ensuring expansion of quality DOTS services to the entire country. There were many challenges remaining that needed to be addressed to achieve the TB-related targets set by the Millennium Development Goals for 2015 and to achieve TB control in the longer term.

The RNTCP has now entered its second phase in which the programme aims to firstly consolidate the gains made to date, to widen services both in terms of activities and access, and to sustain the achievements for decades to come in order to achieve ultimate objective of TB control in the country.

All components of new Stop TB Strategy are incorporated in the second phase of RNTCP. These are:

- Pursue quality DOTS expansion and enhancement, by improving the case finding and cure through an effective patient-centred approach to reach all patients, especially the poor.
- Address TB-HIV, MDR-TB and other challenges, by scaling up TB-HIV joint activities, DOTS Plus, and other relevant approaches.
- Contribute to health system strengthening, by collaborating with other health programmes and general services.
- Involve all health care providers, public, non-governmental and private, by scaling up approaches based on a public-private mix (PPM), to ensure adherence to the International Standards of TB care.
- Engage people with TB, and affected communities to demand, and contribute to effective care. This would involve scaling-up of community TB care; creating demand thorugh context-specific advocacy, communication and social mobilization.

- Enable and promote research for the development of new drugs, diagnostic techniques and vaccines. Research was also needed to improve programme performance.

The Revised National TB Control Programme now aims to widen the scope for providing standardized, good quality treatment and diagnostic services to all TB patients in a patient-friendly environment, in every health care facility they seek treatment from. Recognizing the need to reach every TB patient in the country, the programme has made special provisions to reach marginalized sections of the society, including creating demand for services through specific advocacy, communication and social mobilization activities.

Involvement of other Sectors

Non-Governmental Organizations (NGOs) and Private Practitioners (PP)

Along with a widely available public sector health services in the country, the private health sector operating through NGOs and private health service providers forms an important source of health care. It is believed that the private sector health facilities are often closer to and more trusted by patients and perform an active role in health promotion in the community. Accordingly, RNTCP recognized the need for their involvement to create an epidemiological impact of Tuberculosis control. Thus, public private mix (PPM) under RNTCP was designed with the aim to create an effective link between the national TB programme and all public and private health care providers presently out of realms of national TB programme efforts so as to provide standardized treatment to all TB patients in the country. The Government of India provided guidelines for this link in 2000 and 2001 respectively. However, realizing the importance of the link the latest guidelines effective 1st October 2008 have been issued[2]. The need for revision was felt because of several reasons, including the following:

[2]Revised National Tuberculosis Control Programme, Revised Schemes for NGOs and Private Providers, Central TB Division, Directorate General of Health Services Ministry of Health and Family Welfare, Nirman Bhavan, New Delhi 110108, August 2008.
http://www.tbcindia.org.

- Newer initiatives like DOTS plus.
- TB- HIV collaboration to improve the access of DOTS for the TB patients.
- Emergence of Multidrug resistant TB challenging the RNTCP implementation.
- Long duration of treatment requiring social support network to facilitate adherence to ambulatory treatment.
- Need to provide DOTS services in urban slums to special groups like migrants and slum dwellers.

In 2008, the participation of this sector was considerable with a support of over 2500 NGOs, 25000 PPs, 260 Medical colleges and 150 corporate houses which were providing DOTS services.

The current guidelines have identified the following areas for the collaboration of NGOs and other private collaborators[3].

- TB advocacy, communication, and social mobilization (ACSM Scheme).
- Sputum collection centre/s (SC Scheme).
- Sputum pick-up and transport service (transport scheme).
- Designated microscopy cum treatment centre (A and B) (DMC Scheme).
- Strengthening RNTCP diagnostic services (LT scheme).
- Providing quality assured culture and drug susceptibility testing services (culture and DST scheme).
- Promoting treatment adherence (adherence scheme).
- Improving TB control in urban slums (slum scheme).
- Tuberculosis Unit Model.
- Delivering TB-HIV interventions to high HIV Risk groups (HRGs) (TB-HIV scheme).

The guidelines also give detailed description of eligibility criteria to be satisfied by collaborating agents, their role vis-a vis-RNTCP and financial provisions for carrying out specified activities. They stipulate that private players will act in consultation with relevant Government agencies such as District TB Officer, State TB Officer and District Health Society, for effective and unified out put of the programme.

[3]Ibid.

TB/HIV coordination activities: Since active TB disease is the commonest opportunistic infection amongst HIV-infected individuals, RNTCP has been designed to take care of this situation. The use of low cost and highly effective DOTS strategy of diagnosis and treatment for TB nationwide has been effective for treating TB patients with or without HIV infection. The work related to control and management of HIV is done under the auspices of National Aids Control Organization (NACO). The collaboration between the two establishments is considered necessary to manage the deadly combination of the double infection. TB-HIV collaborative activities started initially in the year 2001, in the six states with high prevalence of HIV/AIDS, i.e. Andhra Pradesh, Karnataka, Maharashtra, Manipur, Nagaland and Tamil Nadu. These activities were extended to eight additional States of Delhi, Gujarat, Himachal Pradesh, Kerala, Orissa, Punjab, Rajasthan and West Bengal in the year 2004 and to entire country in 2007-08, and became an integral part of NACP III (National AIDS Control Programme III) and RNTCP II[4]. The National Framework, in this context, aims to achieve reduced burden of TB and HIV in India through enhanced collaboration between RNTCP and NACP. Its objectives include:

- To establish mechanisms for coordination between RNTCP and NACP at National, State and District levels.
- To decrease morbidity and mortality due to tuberculosis among persons living with HIV/AIDS; and
- To decrease the impact of HIV in tuberculosis patients and provide access to HIV related care and support to HIV-infected TB patients.

Key activities identified under TB/HIV coordination include:

- Establishment of coordination mechanisms at national, state and district level.
- Service delivery coordination and cross-referrals, through training of the programme officials and the field staff and

[4]National Framework for JOINT TB/HIV Collaborative Activities, February 2008, Central TB Division and National AIDS Control Organization, Ministry of Health and Family Welfare, Government of India, New Delhi.

establishment of linkages between service delivery sites of NACP and RNTCP diagnostic and treatment services.
- Involvement of NGOs working in NACP and RNTCP in TB/HIV collaborative activities.
- Operational research to improve the implementation of TB/HIV collaborative activities; and
- Implementation of feasible and effective infection control measures.

Establishment of Collaborative Mechanisms at National, State and District Level

The mechanism set for collaborative activities at national, state and district levels are as follows:

National level: A National Technical Working Group (TWG) has been established to review, optimize, plan and supervise TB/HIV coordination activities in the country. It comprises of key officials from NACO, CTD dealing with TB/HIV Collaborative activities and WHO.

State level: (1) State coordination committees: The committee is chaired by Principal Health Secretary. It ensures smooth implementation and regular review of TB/HIV programmes. The collaborative activities include sending reports to NACO and CTD.

(2) State technical working group (STWG): The Group includes key officials from SACS (PD and APD) and State TB Cell (STO, second MO if present), along with other officials dealing with TB/HIV collaborative activities and consultants working with both the programmes. The State TWG would review and streamline the collaborative activities. In these monthly meetings of TWG, apart from a review of the on-going TB/HIV collaborative activities, the key issues emerging from the district coordination meetings and the cross-referral reports are to be discussed. Based on the discussions, feedback should be sent to the districts on their performance and identified issues. Follow up action taken should be monitored and minutes of the meetings forwarded to NACO and CTD. Every quarter at least one district should be jointly visited by officials from STC and SACS. The observations made in these joint field visits should be submitted in a report to NACO and CTD, and discussed in the State level review meetings.

District level: A District Coordination Committee will ensure smooth implementation and regular review of TB/HIV Collaborative activities, meet on a quarterly basis and send the report to SACS and State TB Cell.

Monthly meeting at the District level involving the DTO and the DNO should be held with the participation of key staff from both the programmes. During these monthly key staff meetings, additional session be organized for TB/HIV which should be attended by the key district staff of NACP. In these monthly meetings a review of the on-going TB/HIV collaborative activities and discussion on key issues emerging from the field should be done. Based on the discussions, feedback should be sent to the service delivery centres on their performance and on any identified issues. Follow-up action taken should be monitored and minutes of the meetings forwarded to SACS and STC.

RNTCP conducts regular programme reviews at the National and State levels. It is planned that at one of these reviews at the National level, an annual review of the TB/HIV Collaborative activities would be held with the participation of State programme managers of both programmes. The annual review would be held in close coordination between NACO and CTD. Similar annual reviews would be held at the State level by adding an additional day to one of the quarterly RNTCP review meetings and inviting the district Nodal officers for HIV/AIDS and SACS officials. These State level reviews are to be organized in coordination with SACS and STC. Whenever possible representatives from CTD and NACO would be attending these State reviews.

To facilitate coordination and successful implementation of TB/HIV collaborative activities, the following positions have been sanctioned:

- A full-time regular government officer in-charge of TB/HIV Collaborative activities in the programmes at the National and State level in NACP and RNTCP. Additional technical support has been provided by RNTCP in form of 2 WHO RNTCP Consultants for TB/HIV collaborative activities at the National level (One at NACO and one at CTD).

- High HIV-Prevalence States: Medical Consultants for TB/HIV have been sanctioned by NACP (for SACS) in Andhra Pradesh, Karnataka, Maharashtra, Tamil Nadu, Nagaland and Manipur.
- *Additional states:* TB/HIV Coordinators have been sanctioned by RNTCP in Assam, Bihar, Chhattisgarh, Delhi, Gujarat, Himachal Pradesh, Jharkhand, Kerala, Madhya Pradesh, Orissa, Punjab, Rajasthan, Uttar Pradesh, Uttaranchal and West Bengal.

Service delivery coordination and cross referral: Following provisions are in place for implementing this component of the programme.

All Settings

- Training of programme officials and field staff on TB/HIV.
- Intensified TB Case Finding at ICTCs, ART Centres, and Care and Support Centres.
- Risk-based referral of TB patients for voluntary HIV counselling and testing.
- Referral of HIV-infected TB patients to NACP for additional care and support, including antiretroviral treatment.

Intensified TB/HIV Package of Services

- Routine referral of all TB patients for HIV counselling and testing.
- Provision of cotrimoxazole preventative therapy (CPT) to HIV-infected TB patients.
- Expanded recording and reporting.

The periodic HIV survey in TB patients for the year 2006–07 demonstrated a wide distribution of HIV prevalence among TB patients across the country. Central TB Division (CTD) and National AIDS Control Organization (NACO) have adopted the policy of providing an "Intensified TB/HIV package" for States with the highest estimated Sero-prevalence of HIV infection. In RNTCP, policy implementation, training, monitoring, and supervision are primarily state-led activities; to ensure the effective implementation of TB/HIV collaborative activities. Intensified TB/HIV Package would be rolled-out on a state by state basis.

Advocacy, communication and social mobilization and involvement of NGOs working in NACP and RNTCP in TB/HIV collaborative activities: A large number of NGOs working with both NACP and RNTCP play an important role in programme implementation by increasing the out reach of the individual programmes and the provision of a package of services to difficult to reach populations like migrant populations, truck drivers, tribal populations, commercial sex workers, etc. The programme contains the following spectrum of activities that may be undertaken by NGOs.

- Dissemination of HIV prevention information through IEC materials prepared by NACP.
- Condom promotion and awareness regarding prevention of HIV.
- Dissemination of information on TB through RNTCP IEC material.
- Referral of persons with HIV risk factors to ICTCs.
- Referring HIV-infected persons to care and support facilities.
- Intensified TB case finding by regular symptom screening.
- Referral of persons with TB symptoms to RNTCP diagnostic facilities.
- Opening of DMC (where appropriate) or establishing a mechanism for sputum collection and transportation to nearest DMC.
- DOTS provision

Operational Research to Improve the Implementation of TB/HIV Collaborative Activities

The priority areas for collaborative operational research with both programmes for TB/HIV include:

- Piloting mechanisms of provider-initiated routine referral of TB patients for counseling and testing for HIV.

- Improving access to HIV related care and support for TB patients who are found to be HIV-infected.
- Estimating TB burden in various setting providing HIV care, like ICTCs, ART centres, and care and support centres.
- Strengthening referral linkages from ICTCs, Care and Support Centres, and ART centres to RNTCP services.
- Strengthening referral linkages of HIV-infected TB patients from general health services to ART centres.
- Reducing mortality of HIV-infected TB patients during and after TB treatment.
- Evaluating the feasibility, efficacy, and optimal duration of Isoniazid prophylactic therapy for prophylaxis of TB at ART and care and support centres; and
- Development of TB screening guidelines for ART centres and care and support centres.

Infection control practices: This activity includes the following:

- Prevention of spread of TB in facilities caring for HIV-infected persons.
- Prevention of spread of HIV through safe injection practices in facilities providing RNTCP services.

Medical colleges: The RNTCP accepts the importance of the role the medical colleges can play in the programme because large numbers of TB patients are treated at medical college hospitals. Their role is two fold: one in the area of training health personnel and two in the area of providing health services. These colleges help the programme through introduction of the principles of DOTS in the medical curriculum and also serving as advocates of the programme. Consensus workshops have been organized regularly every year since 2001 after the first one held in 1997. These workshops have been instrumental in defining the structure and processes for effective involvement of medical colleges in the RNTCP. As a follow-up to these workshops national, five zonal and state level taskforces and core committees in the medical colleges have been established to monitor the involvement of medical colleges in the respective units. Details of these recommendations are available on the website of the department (http://www.tbcindia.org).

Following the recommendations of national workshop held in October 2002, the RNTCP established nodal centres. Since increasing number of medical colleges were participating in the programme as tuberculosis units, microscopy centers, treatment observation centers, etc. it was found necessary that this partnership between an ever increasing number of medical colleges and the RNTCP was nurtured and carried forward. To this effect it was thought essential to establish RNTCP nodal centers in different zones of the country. Ensuring representations from all zones (North, East, West, South and North-East), and based on Government of India's criteria, the workshop recommended a number of colleges which were given the responsibility to function as nodal centers.

These annual workshops have played an important role in strengthening the RNTCP in several key areas. To have a glimpse of their involvement we may cite the areas where recommendations were made in the latest workshop of National Task Force in October 2007. Each recommendation was complete in giving details about how to go about to achieve the desired results. Some of the key areas, among others, were:

- Role of medical colleges in promoting amongst students and peer faculty the use of ISTC, NTF Consensus Statement on use of second line anti-TB drugs and RNTCP patient management guidelines.
- Effective involvement of all departments of Medical Colleges.
- Operational research activities to be conducted by medical colleges, identification of constraints and recommendations to address the constraints.
- Medical College quarterly reports.
- Role of medical colleges towards strengthening MTb culture and DST network.
- Approach to develop NTF recommendations on prevention and transmission of airborne infection (including TB) in hospital settings.

Some of the details of these recommendations give the extent of the interest of medical colleges in the programme and furthering realization of its objectives.

- Sensitize all faculties, students at various levels, para-medicals, nurses and private health care workers about the programme and its implications in promoting national health.
- Include RNTCP guidelines in prescribed text books for medical students at various level.
- Produce user friendly booklet (similar to "RNTCP at a Glance") on RNTCP DOTS and DOTS Plus to provide guidelines to be made available incorporating ISTC and NTF recommendations on rational usage of second line anti-TB drugs.
- Include all clinical Head of Departments including super specialties in medical college as members in the core committee and hold core committee meetings every quarter as per norms.
- Encourage Operational Research and Thesis work on DOTS.
- Promote advocacy through electronic and print media.
- Train 'master trainers' from medical college faculty with emphasis on the rational use of second line anti-TB drugs to be included.
- Constitute national and state level committees in medical colleges to look into treatment of suspected MDR TB cases.

Training: Sound technical and training policies have been formulated. The RNTCP has developed a number of training modules. The latest available list given below shows the extent of these modules which are constantly revised and up-dated.

Modules

- Addendum on REVISED RECORDING and REPORTING FORMATS – March 2008.
- DST-DRS Training Manual RNTCP.
- Managing the RNTCP in your area—a training course (Modules 1–4).

- Managing the RNTCP in your area—A training course (Modules 5–9).
- Training module for medical practitioners.
- Module for Senior Tuberculosis Laboratory Supervisors.
- Module for Senior Treatment Supervisors.
- Financial Management Training Module.
- Module for laboratory technicians.
- Training Manual for DTC Drug Store.
- Training Manual for DTC Drug Store (Solutions to Exercises).
- Module for MPWs and other DOT Providers.
- Improving Interpersonal Communication.
- Guide for Course Directors and Facilitators.
- RNTCP at a Glance.

TB/HIV

- Training Module for Counsellors on TB/HIV Coordination.
- Training Module for Medical Officers on TB/HIV.
- Training Module for STS and STLS on TB/HIV Coordination.

Training Manuals for Intensified TB/HIV Package

- For Program Managers at State and District Level
- For Medical Officers
- For Pharmacists
- For ICTC Counsellors

Exercise Books

- Managing the RNTCP in your area—A training course (Exercise Workbook E1-Laboratory Forms, E2-Treatment Cards, E3-TB Register and E1-3 Answer Guide).
- Module for Senior Treatment Supervisors–Exercise Workbook.

3

Incidence and Prevalence

"Five thousand people (globally) die from tuberculosis every day, although the disease is both preventable and curable. Clearly, we must work harder if we are to achieve by 2015, the Millennium Development Goal of halting and beginning to reverse the spread of TB as one of the world's major diseases".

Kofi Annan UN Secretary General

"For this prolonged struggle towards achieving TB control in India, the highest levels of commitment are required from the states to maintain and improve the quality of DOTS services provided to our citizens".

Dr. Anbumani Ramadoss, 2006
Minister of Health and Family Welfare, Govt. of India

3.1 INTRODUCTION

The infectious nature and wide prevalence of the disease has remained one of the most serious concerns of the humanity ever since the civilization began. Scientists have been busy all the time in battling against tuberculosis and striving to get control over it. The two basic requirements for achieving success in this endeavor have remained the assessment of the extent of the disease and the development of techniques to control and eradicate it. The present chapter summarizes the extent of the disease in India as compared to selected countries, the regions and in the world at large. It also presents the measurement of intensity of tuberculosis in India along with differentials in burden by administrative divisions of the country. Here we have reviewed the data mainly from the official sources and the population based surveys available in India with reference to various time periods. We attempt to validate these data and arrive at some plausible estimates of the extent of the disease in the country. To arrive at comparative picture in other areas we have largely taken the statistics from publications of WHO. The status of various strategies for controlling and eradicating the disease in the country is taken up in chapter four.

3.2 EXTENT OF TUBERCULOSIS

Tuberculosis presently, is one of the most deadly and common major infectious diseases afflicting the world's population. In 2007, there were an estimated number of about 9.273 million (139 per 100,000 persons) new cases of TB (all forms) including 4.062 million (44% of the total) or 62 per 100,000 persons of new smear-positive cases[1]. The number of TB patients in the World in that year was estimated at 13.723 million or 206 per 100,000 persons, about 0.7 million fewer than 14.4 million cases in 2006. About 1.772 million (1.316 HIV negative and 0.456 HIV positive) died of TB in the same year. The corresponding rates were 20 and 7 per 100,000 persons per year. These estimates were, as expected, much higher than the number of notified cases compiled from the reports submitted by 196 of the 208 countries reporting to WHO. These countries together notified only 5.572 million new and relapse cases of which 2.581 million (46%) were new smear-positive. These figures include 5.490 million new and relapsed cases from DOTS areas including 2.557 million new smear-positive cases. In 13 years since 1995 DOTS areas notified altogether 37.3 million new and relapsed cases and 18.1 million new smear-positive cases. Among the new cases around 709,000 (7.7%) were HIV-positive cases. The new smear – positive notified cases were only 56% of the estimated incidence of such cases. India, China, Indonesia, Nigeria, and South Africa rank first to fifth respectively in terms of absolute numbers of cases. The African Region has the highest incidence rate of 363 per 100,000 persons.

The estimated incidence, prevalence and mortality for all forms of TB in India in 2007 were 1.962 million, 3.305 million and

[1]WHO: Global Tuberculosis Control 2009: Epidemiology, Strategy, Financing. WHO Report 2009, Geneva, World Health Organization (Table 1.2). This report uses the latest data available.

0.332 million, respectively, giving the corresponding rates of 168, 283 and 28.5 per 100,000 persons per year. The incidence of smear-positive cases was 0.873 million or 75 per 100,000 persons. Like the global figures, the number of notified cases fell short of the estimates. The notification of all new and relapse cases was slightly more than 1.296 million and of new smear positive cases was about 0.593 million or slightly more than 60% of the estimate[2]. Among the new cases about 1.2% was HIV-positive.

Based on WHO data for 2007 all forms of TB in India accounted for almost 21% of the estimated TB burden in the world. Somewhat similar (22%) share is for new smear-positive cases. As far as prevalence of and mortality caused by TB are concerned, India accounted for about 24% and 19% of the world's burden. India ranked at number one in TB burden, among 196 countries that comprised the WHO data base for 2007. For comparative purposes, it may be noted that China, with much larger population base than India, ranked at number 2 with substantially lower TB burden: the incidence, prevalence and mortality burden for all forms of TB in China were, respectively, about 14%, 19% and 11% of the world burden. The respective figures for burdens of TB in India were about 50%, 28% and 65% higher than that in China. Even the incidence of new smear-positive cases of TB in India was about 49% higher than that in China.

It may be pointed out here that WHO ranks the countries for TB burden according to the number of incident cases from highest to lowest. On this scaling 22 countries (11 in Asia, 9 in Africa, one each in Latin America and Russian Federation) have been identified as High Burden Countries (HBCs). Of these the burden in India is the highest at 1.962 million and that in Afghanistan is lowest at 0.06 million. Of the top ten HBCs, six (India, China, Indonesia, Bangladesh, Pakistan and Philippines) are in Asia and the remaining four (Nigeria, South Africa, Ethiopia and DR Congo) are in Africa.

An alternative way of examining the status of TB is through the measurement of the intensity of the disease. This can be done by normalizing the incident cases in terms of population size and expressed in unit of 100,000 persons per year. We may

[2]WHO op. cit.

define the intensity of the disease with the help of such normalized rates of incidence, prevalence and mortality. These normalized rates show that only China, Russian Federation, Brazil, Thailand and Afghanistan with respective incident rates for all form of TB at 99, 107, 50, 142 and 161 showed lower incident rates than that in India in 2006. A comparative picture of the intensity of TB in India and selected countries and regions is given in Table 3.1. Appendix Table 3.1 at the end of the chapter presents the detailed data for high burden countries and different regions of the world as available from WHO source for the year 2007. It may be noted from Table 3.1 that of the three neighbouring countries, two Bangladesh and Pakistan have higher incident rates than that for India. The highest incident rate per 100,000 persons per year was noted for South

Table 3.1: Estimated intensity of TB, India, selected high burden countries and regions, 2006

Country/Region	*Rates per 100,000 Persons per year*				*HIV Prev. in incident TB cases (%)*
	Incidence		*Prevalence*	*Mortality*	
	All Forms	*Smear-positive*	*All Forms*	*All Forms*	
India	168	75	299	28	1.2
Neighbouring areas					
China	99	45	201	15	0.3
Bangladesh	225	101	391	45	0.0
Pakistan	181	82	263	34	0.3
South Africa	940	382	998	218	44
Kenya	384	153	334	72	52
Zimbabwe	557	227	597	131	43
Cambodia	500	220	665	92	9.6
Brazil	50	31	55	4.0	12
All HBCs	177	79	286	32	11
SEAR	180	81	289	30	1.3
Global	139	62	219	25	7.7

Source: Global Tuberculosis Control: surveillance, planning, financing. WHO report 2008. Geneva, World Health Organization, Table 1.2.

Note: HBC: High Burden Country, SEAR: South East Asia Region.

Africa (940) which was followed by Zimbabwe (557) and Cambodia (500). Other rates showed similar trend.

A summary giving level of prevalence of TB in India estimated by different sources and reference years is given in Table 3.2. The table also gives the estimated number of TB cases in India in 2006 with reference to prevalence rate estimated by different sources. It may be noted that the National Family Health Survey and WHO provide the prevalence rate for all forms of tuberculosis. By contrast, Indian Council of Medical Research figure refers to sputum positive cases only and therefore is expected to be lower than that for all forms of the disease. The last column of Table 3.2 is meant only to illustrate the TB burden in India if the rates given by various sources were in operation in 2006. This exercise shows that the burden of tuberculosis might be as low as 3.5 million or as high as 6.4 million.

Since tuberculosis affects the working population mostly and thus impacting the economic productivity, its adverse implication to business could not be ignored. In this context business leaders across the globe at World Economic Forum in 2008 agreed that tuberculosis posed one of the gratest silent threats to the private sector and needed to be tackled on a war footing if people of prime working age between 15 and 54 years, particularly in fast-growing developing countries, were not to succumb to the disease[3]. The WEF report pointed to the fact that nearly one-third of over 11,000 business leaders from more than 130 countries expected TB to affect their business in the next five years. The report said that companies in Asia, sub-Saharan Africa and Eastern Europe were most concerned and those in countries like India, which were additionally hard hit by AIDS, were particularly worried about TB.

3.3 MEASUREMENT OF INCIDENCE AND PREVALENCE OF TUBERCULOSIS IN INDIA

The information about incidence, prevalence and associated mortality are the important elements of the study of the extent of any disease, including tuberculosis, in the population. The

[3]'TB silent threat to working people', Times of India, Delhi, March 23, 2008.

Table 3.2: Estimates of prevalence rate of tuberculosis per 100,000 persons for all India by source and reference year along with estimated burden of the disease in 2006

Source	*Reference year*	*Prevalence rate 100,000 persons per year*	*Estimated number of TB cases in India in 2006 ('000)*
Indian Council of Medical Research (ICMR)	1955–58	400*	4,456
National Family Health Survey – 1st Round	1992–93	467**	5,202
National Family Health Survey – 2nd Round	1998–99	544**	6,060
National Family Health Survey – 3rd Round	2005–06	445**	4,957
WHO	1990	570***	6,350
	2004	312***	3,476
	2006	299***	3,331

Notes:

* *The figure refers to sputum positive TB.*

** *The figure refers to all forms of TB as reported in the survey.*

*** *Refers to all forms of TB.*

The estimated number of TB cases in 2006 has been obtained by combining the prevalence rate and the estimated population of India in 2006 at 1,114 million.

associated rates in conjunction with total population provide the numerical burden of the disease. Data on incidence, measuring the occurrence of the number of new cases in a year, are required to predict the burden of any disease including tuberculosis. However important, it is extremely difficult to assess the incidence of *M. tuberculosis* infections in a community because, in the absence of spontaneous response and reporting and reluctance in health seeking behaviour of the patients, this requires repeated tuberculosis tests in large samples of population that has to be interpreted for boosting and reversion. In addition, there are problems with the receiver operating characteristic curve (ROC) of the test where the assessment of discriminating the healthy and the diseased person is done. Therefore, this is generally estimated indirectly[4]. World Health Organization (WHO) has given a number of definitions that link most of the required parameters for the assessment of the extent of the disease in the community or in any large population group[5]. These relate incidence of the disease to the other parameters needed for its computation. Among these, the incidence of the disease is the key parameter which needs to be estimated. In India this estimation is done presently using the Annual Risk of Tuberculosis Infection (ARTI) defined as the probability of acquiring new infection during the course of one year. This is computed from the estimated prevalence of infection among younger children and it is the first epidemiological parameter to be affected following a change in the tuberculosis situation in the community. Also, it emulated the

---

[4]Dipanjan Roy, LS Chauhan, Epidemiology of Tuberculosis in SP Agarwal and LS Chauhan, (Eds.) (2005): Tuberculosis Control in India, Directorate General of Health Services, Ministry of Health and Family Welfare, New Delhi.

[5]WHO Report 2006 on Global Tuberculosis Control: Surveillance, Planning, Financing, gives four definitions to link various measures of TB as follows:

Incidence = Case notifications/Proportion of cases detected
Incidence = Prevalence/Duration of Condition of disease
Incidence = Annual Risk of Infection* Styblo co-efficient
Incidence = Deaths/Proportion of incident cases that die

The Styblo co-efficient is taken to be a constant, with an empirically derived value in the range 40 – 60 relating Annual Risk of Tuberculosis Infection (%) to incidence of smear-positive cases (per 1000,000 per year).

overall impact of various factors influencing the transmission of tubercle bacilli such as prevalence of infectious cases in the community and efficiency of case finding and treatment activity. The ARTI is an algebraically derived probability of tuberculosis infection calculated from the prevalence of infection at a given age[6].

Risk of Infection and Infectious Cases

The risk of infection in the community during a period (usually one year) depends upon the number of successful transmissions from infectious cases to susceptible individuals. In the case of tuberculosis it is estimated that one infectious case, on the average, infects about 10–15 new cases every year. For the pre-chemotherapeutic era, it was estimated by Karel Styblo, that one infectious case infected about 20 new cases every two years, the period of infectivity before either spontaneous conversion or death of the case. He further assumed that the lifetime risk of developing infectious or sputum-positive TB following infection with TB bacilli to be 5 percent. Thus, knowing the annual risk of tuberculosis infection, the incidence of infectious TB can be obtained as 5% of the ARTI. Taken for a base of 100,000 persons, if the ARTI is 1%, it will mean that there will be 1000 persons likely to be infected. Of this 5% or 50 (1000 × 0.5) will be sputum-positive or infectious. In India the estimated incidence of infectious TB cases per year is 75 per 100,100 persons which correspond to ARTI of 1.5 percent.

Estimation of ARTI in India

Epidemiological situation of tuberculosis needs to be studied in order to have baseline data and to formulate strategies and to see the impact of such strategies for control of tuberculosis.

---

[6]The formula for calculation of ARTI is as follows.
$Rx + a/2 = 1 - (1 - Px + a)\ 1/a$.
where $Rx + a/2$ = Annual Risk of infection at the midpoint in the calendar time between the year the cohort was born (x^0) and the year of the survey, i.e. the age of the cohort (a).
$Px + a$ = Prevalence rate of infection at the time of survey, Each rate is expressed on the unit base, i.e. it is a fraction, and x – is the midpoint of the calendar year the cohort was born and a is the midpoint of the age group for which the prevalence rate is estimated.

Various epidemiological indicators like tuberculin test, chest X-ray, sputum examination and mortality rate, etc. have been used in the past to study the epidemiological situation. However, in the given scenario of high prevalence of tuberculosis and large population these methods are found to be expensive and time consuming. Annual risk of infection (ARI) is one epidemiological index which has been found to be useful to study the epidemiological situation because it is easy to perform and is cost effective. However, there is controversy about the study of ARI in BCG vaccinated children. In the era of universal immunization program (UIP) it is very difficult to find sufficient number of non BCG vaccinated children. Therefore ARI was estimated amongst BCG vaccinated and non BCG vaccinated children.

National Level ARTI Surveys

In view of the importance of ARTI in any programme directed towards tuberculosis control, lack of any reliable data for the entire country and the cost involved in collecting data, the government of India implemented the conduct of a nation-wide tuberculosis survey during 2000–03, at a time when the tuberculosis control activities were being intensified under the RNTCP. The objective of the survey was to estimate the prevalence of infection among children one to nine years of age and to compute average ARTI in each of the four defined zones into which the country was stratified for the purpose of the survey. The survey was conducted independently in each zone (north, south, east and west) following a uniform methodology, with NTI (National TB Institute, Bangalore) as the nodal centre and TRC (TB Research Centre), Chennai, as the collaborating centre with local support from state health authorities. Two different methods, were used to estimate the prevalence of tuberculosis infection[7]. The results are presented in Table 3.3.

[7]VK Chadha, SP Agarwal, LS Chauhan, Annual Risk of Tuberculosis Infection in Different Zones of India. In SP Agarwal and LS Chauhan, (Eds.) (2005) : Tuberculosis Control in India, Directorate General of Health Services, Ministry of Health and Family Welfare, New Delhi.

Table 3.3: Estimated prevalence of infection (PI) and annual risk of tuberculosis infection (ARTI) by zones, India, 2000–03.

	Method I				Method II			
	PI (%)			*ARTI (%)*	*PI (%)*			*ARTI (%)*
Zone	*Rural*	*Urban*	*Total*	*Total*	*Rural*	*Urban*	*Total*	*Total*
North	9.1	14.1	10.3	1.9	8.2	17.4	10.5	1.9
South	4.5	9.8	6.1	1.1	4.7	8.8	5.9	1.0
West	7.8	12.6	9.3	1.8	7.4	10.99	8.5	1.6
East	6.5	9.0	6.9	1.3	6.5	8.3	6.9	1.3

ARTI for all India was estimated as 1.5 percent.

Source: Annual Risk of Tuberculosis Inspection in Different Zones of Inida, A National Sample Survey, 2000–2003 by VK Chadha, SP Agarwal, LS Chauhan given in Tuberculosis Control in India, SP Agarwal and LS Chauhan, Director General of Health Service, Ministry of Health and Family welfare, New Delhi, 2005.

The values of ARTI given in Table 7.3 and the Styblo coefficient of 5% applied to the relevant equation given by WHO[8] yield the estimate for the number of new smear-positive pulmonary TB cases. For example for ARTI of 1.5 percent per year as estimated for India, there are 75 cases per 100,000 persons who are expected to be smear-positive for pulmonary tuberculosis.

Using ARTI estimates at zonal level, CTD (Central TB Division, Directorate General of Health Services, Ministry of Health and Family Welfare, Government of India) has given the estimated number for incidence of new smear-positive TB cases per 100,000 persons in the year 2003 for north, east, south and west zones as 95, 75, 75, and 80. The estimate of incidence rate for Orissa was given as 85 per 100, 000 persons and it was taken out of the east zone for estimation purpose. The incidence rates for 2004 and 2005 in the four zones remained at the level for 2003. The incidence rates for earlier two years, 2001 and 2002 were 50, 115, 100 and 85 for Kerala, Himachal Pradesh, Manipur and the rest of the country respectively.

According to ARTI survey (2000–03) the tuberculosis situation in most parts of India appeared grave with an average of 1,100–1,900 persons in different zones out of every 100,000

[8]Incidence = ARTI* Styblo Coefficient, see footnote 1.

acquiring new tuberculosis infection each year of which 50 to 95 per 100,000 persons were likely to get smear-positive. Another observation worth concern was that TB situation in urban areas was worse than in rural areas. This aspect is examined in detail in Section 3.5.

In view of the importance of the estimate of ARTI in TB control programme, India launched the second large-scale country-wide study to ascertain the number of people who fall prey to tuberculosis every year. This next round of ARTI survey to be carried out during 2007–2009, beginning January 2007, is to cover about 300,000 children which is about 50% larger than that in the first round of the survey. The findings are expected to provide the clearer picture of the effectiveness of the TB control programme implemented through DOTS strategy currently in use. The survey, like the earlier one, will be conducted by the Tuberculosis Research Centre, Chennai and the National Tuberculosis Institute, Bengaluru[9]. The findings of the survey, hopefully, will improve our understanding of the incidence of tuberculosis noted in the first ARTI survey.

Localized ARTI Surveys

A number of small scale localized surveys have been conducted in the past to estimate the annual risk of infection for tuberculosis. Some of these are mentioned here.

- A sample of 4053 children in the district of Patiala was used to estimate the annual risk of infection for tuberculosis. The study revealed[10] that the prevalence rate of tuberculosis was 7.01% (7.54% females, 6.74% males). The prevalence of tuberculin positivity in BCG vaccinated and non BCG vaccinated children was 7.22% and 6.68% respectively. The estimated annual risk of infection was 1.12 in all the groups. No statistical difference was observed between rural/urban, BCG/non BCG vaccinated, and male/female subjects.

---

[9]Times of India, Delhi Edition, September 27, 2006.

[10]Jai Kishan, MBBS, BK Kapoor and Rohit K Singla, Estimation of Annual Risk of Infection of Tuberculosis in District Patiala, INDIA, 2003 by the American College of Chest Physicians., Mycobacterial Infection: US and International Perspectives, Wednesday, October 29, 2003.

- A survey of rural and urban areas of eight selected districts in the state of Orissa, India[11] was carried out to estimate the average annual risk of tuberculosis infection (ARTI) in the state. A community-based, cross-sectional tuberculin survey was conducted among 10,626 children aged 1–9 years. A stratified sampling was adopted for selection of clusters. Highly trained designated tuberculin testers administered 0.1 ml (1 TU) of PPD RT 23 with Tween 80 by the Mantoux method to 10,626 children. Transverse tuberculin reaction sizes were measured about 72 hrs. later by trained designated tuberculin readers. The number of children satisfactorily test-read was 10,191. Based on the frequency distribution of tuberculin reaction sizes, the average ARTI in the state was estimated at 1.7–1.8%. The children residing in urban areas were observed to be at a significantly higher risk of infection than those in rural areas.
- The Annual Risk of Tuberculosis Infection in Bangalore City[12] was carried out to assess the existing epidemiological situation of tuberculosis and to provide baseline information for assessment of trends in the future. The survey was conducted in 161 schools located in Bangalore city, from February 1996 to February 1999. A single stage cluster sampling design was adopted for the selection of schools by simple random sampling. The universe was defined by a consolidated list of 1,780 Govt.-run, Govt. aided and Private schools. The selected schools were spread uniformly all over the city. The sample consisted of children aged 6 and 7 years attending these schools. The analysis based on the frequency distribution of reaction sizes among 9,4340 test-read children revealed that 11.1% were estimated to be infected with tubercle bacilli. The children studying in Government-run

[11]AN. Shashidhara, VK Chadha, PS Jagannatha, TK Ray, RN Mania, The Annual risk of Tuberculous Infection in Orissa State, India, International Journal of tuberculosis and Lung Diseases, 8 (5): 545–551.

[12]VK Chadha1, PS Jagannatha and Shashidhar J Savanur, The Annual Risk of Tuberculosis Infection in Bangalore City, Indian Journal of Tuberculosis, 2001, 48, 63–71. *Paper also presented at the 55th National Conference on Tuberculosis and Chest Diseases held In Calcutta, 7–10 December, 2000.

and Government-aided schools were more likely to be infected than those attending private schools. The ARTI in Bangalore city was estimated to be 1.67%. It was higher than the contemporary estimates obtained from the surrounding peri-urban and rural areas. Thus, suggesting a need for further improving the efficiency of case-finding and treatment activities. The results further indicate that BCG vaccinated children can be included for the purpose of estimating ARTI.

- A community-based cross-sectional tuberculin survey among children aged 1–9 years was carried out in the tribal population of Madhya Pradesh, central India[13]. It used a multistage stratified cluster sampling design to select a representative random sample of villages inhabited predominantly by tribal population in selected districts. A total of 4,802 children were tuberculin-tested and the reaction sizes read after 72 hrs. The findings revealed a total of 3,062 (64%) children had no BCG scar. The frequency distribution of children by reaction sizes indicated a fair mode at 18 mm in the right hand side of the distribution. By mirror-image technique, the prevalence of infection among children with no recognizable BCG scar was estimated as 6.8%. The 95% confidence interval for the estimate was 4.8% to 8.9%. The related annual risk of tuberculosis infection was computed as 1.3%, with 95% confidence limit between 0.9% and 1.7%. The corresponding estimates of ARTIs for children irrespective of scar status were 7.1% and 1.3%, with respective 95% confidence limits as 5.5% to 8.8% and 1.0 to 1.7%. The survey revealed that the risk of tuberculosis infection in tribal population of Madhya Pradesh was similar to that in other areas of the country.
- Literature exists on some other area studies which were carried out as a part of the all India study for estimating

[13]VG Rao , PG Gopi, R Yadav , R Subramani , J Bhat, AR Anvikar , K Sadacharam , BK Tiwari, V Gadge , MK Bhondeley, G P Shukla , M Ukey , S Jain and DF Wares, Annual risk of tuberculosis infection among tribal population of central India, Tropical Medicine and International Health, Volume 13, Issue 11, Novermber 2008, pp. 1372–1377.

ARTI cited earlier on. Two such articles are mentioned here[14]. The survey was carried out in a representative sample of villages and census enumeration blocks of towns in four south Indian states, as a part of a nationwide tuberculin survey. Six districts were selected through systematic random sampling. Four hundred and twenty rural clusters and 180 urban clusters were selected from these districts on the basis of the rural-urban ratio in the entire zone. To obtain the required sample of 12,000 children without BCG vaccination, 51,000 had to be covered. Eighty-five children from each cluster were tuberculin tested and read for reaction sizes. The ARTI was computed from the estimated prevalence of TB infection among children without a BCG scar. It was estimated that among 52,951 children registered for the study, 50,846 (96%) had a tuberculin test result. The BCG coverage for the study population was about 65%. Among 17,811 children without a BCG scar, the prevalence of infection was 5.9% (95% CI 4.0–7.7%); the corresponding ARTI was 1.7% (95% CI 0.7–1.4%). The estimated ARTI for the south zone was 1.0%, as compared to the national average of 1.7% used for programme evaluation. The objective of the second study was to estimate the proportion infected and compute Annual Risk of Tuberculosis Infection (ARTI) among children irrespective of BCG scar and compare with that among children without BCG scar. The prevalence of infection and ARTI estimated among children irrespective of BCG scar aged 1–9 years were 5.7% and 1.0% respectively. The corresponding figures among unvaccinated children were 5.9% and 1.0% respectively. The ARTI among children irrespective of BCG scar were similar to that among unvaccinated children.

---

[14](a) Kolappan C, Gopi PG, Subramani R, Chadha VK, Kumar P, Venkatesh Prasad V, Appegowda BN, Nagabhushana Rao RS, Sashidharan R, Ganesan N, Santha T, Narayanan PR, *Estimation of annual risk of tuberculosis infection (ARTI) among children aged 1 – 9 years in the south zone of India,* The International Journal of Tuberculosis and Lung Diseases, Volume 8, Number 4, April 2004, pp. 418 – 423 (6). (b) PG Gopi, R Subramani, C Kolappan, V Venkatesh Prasad and PR Narayanan, *Estimation of Annual Risk of Tuberculosis Infection Among Children Irrespective of BCG Scar in the South Zone of India* Indian J Tuberc 2006; 53: 7-11].

3.4 PREVALENCE OF TUBERCULOSIS IN INDIA AND STATES: HOUSEHOLD SURVEY DATA

There is limited experience in collecting large scale morbidity data through population based demographic surveys in India. However, an attempt was made in National Family Health Survey-First Round conducted during 1992–93 (NHFS-1), to collect data on five major morbidity conditions including tuberculosis[15]. During the field work of the survey, the household head or other knowledgeable adult in the household reported morbidity condition for each household member. No effort was made to do clinical tests for the disease condition. Since the results relating to prevalence of tuberculosis in particular from the survey were found to be generally plausible, the question on morbidity was retained in the subsequent rounds of the National Family Health Survey – Second Round conducted during 1998–99 (NFHS-2)[16] and Third Round conducted during 2005–06 (NFHS-3)[17]. To improve the understanding of the extent of prevalence of tuberculosis in the population in the country and its various regions, NHFS-2 and NFHS-3 expanded the question on tuberculosis to cover the prevalence of medically treated TB along with that reported as in NFHS-1. NFHS-3 conducted during 2005–06 provides data on prevalence of TB in India, comparable to that given by NFHS-2. In addition this round also provides information on knowledge and attitude towards TB.

Based on the three rounds of the National Family Health Survey, Table 3.4 provides information on the prevalence rate (number of persons per 100,000 household population suffering from reported and medically treated tuberculosis) and changes therein by state, India, 1992–93, 1998-99 and 2005–06.

The prevalence of overall tuberculosis in India in 1998–99 at 544 per 100,000 persons was higher than that in 1992–93

[15]National Family Health Survey-1, 1992–93, India, International Institute of Population Sciences, Mumbai.
[16]National Family Health Survey-2, 1998–99, India, International Institute of Population Sciences, Mumbai.
[17]National Family Health Survey-3, 2005–06, India, International Institute of Population Sciences, Mumbai.

Table 3.4: Number of persons per 100,000 household population (prevalence rate) suffering from tuberculosis and changes therein by state, India, 1992-93, 1998–99 and 2005–06

	Prevalence rate					*Percentage change in prevalence rate*			
	Reported cases			*Medically treated*		*Reported cases*			*Med. Tr.*
	NFHS- Rounds								
India/states	**I**	**II**	**III**	**II**	**III**	**I to II**	**II to III**	**I to III**	**II to III**
India	467	544	445	432	418	16.5	–18.2	–4.7	–3.2
North									
Delhi	192	511	240	451	231	166.1	–53.0	25.0	–48.8
Haryana	327	358	340	314	324	9.5	–5.0	4.0	3.2
Himachal Pradesh	242	259	182	234	171	7.0	–29.7	–24.8	–26.9
Jammu & Kashmir*	245	428	104	428	96	74.7	–75.7	–57.6	–77.6
Punjab	238	207	201	197	201	–13.0	–2.9	–15.5	2.0
Rajasthan	724	397	371	342	359	–45.2	–6.5	–48.8	5.0
Uttaranchal	Na	Na	345	Na	329	Na	Na	Na	Na
Central									
Chhattisgarh	Na	Na	310	Na	280	Na	Na	Na	Na
Madhya Pradesh	435	602	353	520	331	38.4	–41.4	–18.9	–36.3
Uttar Pradesh	560	551	450	424	425	–1.6	–18.3	–19.6	0.2

Contd...

Table 3.4: Number of persons per 100,000 household population (prevalence rate) suffering from tuberculosis and changes therein by state, India, 1992-93, 1998–99 and 2005–06 (*Contd...*)

	Prevalence rate					*Percentage change in prevalence rate*			
	Reported cases			*Medically treated*		*Reported cases*			*Med. Tr.*
	NFHS- Rounds								
India/states	**I**	**II**	**III**	**II**	**III**	**I to II**	**II to III**	**I to III**	**II to III**
East									
Bihar	595	989	797	833	735	66.2	–19.4	33.9	–11.8
Jharkhand	Na	Na	659	Na	598	Na	Na	Na	Na
Orissa	555	833	418	707	371	50.1	–49.8	–24.7	–47.5
West Bengal	357	492	605	290	577	37.8	23.0	69.5	99.0
North East									
Arunachal Pradesh	938	1270	1111	1115	1096	35.4	–12.5	18.4	–1.7
Assam	638	710	654	357	605	11.3	–7.9	2.5	69.5
Manipur	951	1107	818	1020	804	16.4	–26.1	–14.0	–21.2
Meghalaya	321	1459	593	648	446	354.5	–59.4	84.7	–31.2
Mizoram	311	1063	528	813	461	241.8	–50.3	69.8	–43.3
Nagaland	491	1654	633	1078	585	236.9	–61.7	28.9	–45.7
Sikkim	Na	Na	613	Na	583	Na	Na	Na	Na

Contd...

Table 3.4: Number of persons per 100,000 household population (prevalence rate) suffering from tuberculosis and changes therein by state, India, 1992-93, 1998–99 and 2005–06 (*Contd...*)

	Prevalence rate					*Percentage change in prevalence rate*			
	Reported cases			*Medically treated*		*Reported cases*			*Med. Tr.*
	NFHS- Rounds								
India/states	**I**	**II**	**III**	**II**	**III**	**I to II**	**II to III**	**I to III**	**II to III**
Tripura	289	1002	647	662	545	246.7	–35.4	123.9	–17.7
West									
Goa	179	466	166	314	166	160.3	–64.4	–7.3	–47.1
Gujarat	308	438	538	357	525	42.2	22.8	74.7	47.1
Maharashtra	293	282	321	230	311	–3.8	13.8	9.6	35.2
South									
Andhra Pradesh	407	592	449	446	409	45.5	–24.2	10.3	–8.3
Karnataka	136	269	141	221	136	97.8	–47.6	3.7	–38.5
Kerala	586	526	275	403	268	–10.2	–47.7	–53.1	–33.5
Tamil Nadu	703	479	508	424	483	–31.9	6.1	–27.7	13.9

* The figure for 1992–93 is for Jammu Region of J and K.
Na: Not available.
Source: Table 8.2 NFHS-1 (1992–93), Table 6.8, NF HS-2 (1998–99), Table 13.2, NFHS-3 (2005-096).

(467) and in 2005–06 (445) by 16 and 22% respectively. Of the 25 states in India, for which data were available, the increase in the prevalence rate during the period 1992–93 to 1998–99 was noted in 19 states. Of the six states which experienced the decline in the prevalence rate, two (Punjab and Rajasthan) were in the north, one (Uttar Pradesh) in the centre, one (Maharashtra) in the west, and 2 (Kerala and Tamil Nadu) in the south. Substantial declines, however, were registered only in two states, Rajasthan in the north (from 724 to 397) and Tamil Nadu in the south (from 703 to 479). The increase in the prevalence rate was quite substantial in most of the states in the north-eastern part of the country. The reported prevalence rate for TB in 1998–99 in the states of Mizoram, Nagaland and Tripura were about three and half times as high as the respective rates in 1992–93. The state of Meghalaya reported even higher rise where the prevalence rate in 1998–99 was four and half times higher than that in 1992–93. Delhi in the north and Goa in the west, with reported prevalence rates in 1992–93 at 192 and 179 respectively, recorded a rise in the prevalence rate as high as two and half times in 1998–99. Karnataka in the south with a prevalence rate 136 in 1992–93 recorded prevalence rate in 1998–99 twice as much as that in 1992–93. Bihar, Orissa, West Bengal in the east; Gujarat in the west; and Andhra Pradesh in the south also showed a rise of about 50% in the prevalence rate during the period covered by the two rounds of the survey.

The period of about seven years that elapsed between NFHS-2 and NFHS-3 witnessed a drop in the prevalence rate for India from 554 per 100,000 persons in 1998–99 to 445 in 2005–06, a drop of about 18%. This drop was more than sufficient to off-set the rise in the prevalence rate during the inter-survey period of rounds one and two. This amounted to a drop of about 5% in the prevalence rate during the period 1992–93 to 2005–06. This feature was shared by many states. As many as twenty one states experienced the fall in the prevalence rate during the inter-survey periods of second and third rounds. The variability in the percentage drop for various states was, however, quite high. All the six states in the north experienced decline which varied between about 3% for Punjab to 76% for Jammu and Kashmir. States in other regions showed lower variability as compared to preceeding states.The decline in the major states was between about 20% and 50%. Only four states (West Bengal in the east, Gujarat and Maharashtra in the west and Tamil Nadu in the south) experienced a rise in the prevalence rate of a magnitude ranging between 6% for Tamil Nadu and 23% for West Bengal and Gujarat).

The prevalence rate in 2005–06 (NFHS-3) was lower than that in 1998–99 in 21 of the 25 states. However, this decline was not large enough to compensate for the rise between 1992–93 and 1998–99 which was noted in 19 states. Only six of these nineteen states, (namely, Himachal Pradesh, Jammu and Kashmir, Madhya Pradesh, Orissa, Manipur, Goa) experienced an overall decline in prevalence rate between 1992–93 and 2005–06. Whereas West Bengal and Gujarat experienced only the rising trend in the prevalence rate, four states, Punjab, Rajasthan, Uttar Pradesh and Kerala experienced the declining trend. The trend of the movement in the prevalence rate over the inter-survey periods is summarized in Table 3.5.

Table 3.5: Pattern of change in prevalence rate for reported tuberculosis in states of India as revealed by data from national family health survey rounds, I (NFHS-I), II (NFHS-II), III (NFHS-III)*.

NFHS rounds			*Names of states*	*Number of states*
I to II	**II to III**	**I to III**		
Increase	Increase	Increase	West Bengal, Gujarat	2
Increase	Decrease	Increase	Delhi, Haryana, Bihar, Arunanchal Pradesh, Assam, Meghalaya, Mizoram Nagaland, Tripura, Andhra Pradesh, Karnataka	11
Increase	Decrease	Decrease	Himachal Pradesh, Jammu & Kashmir, Madhya Pradesh, Orissa, Manipur, Goa	6
Decrease	Increase	Increase	Maharashtra	1
Decrease	Increase	Decrease	Tamil Nadu	1
Decrease	Decrease	Decrease	Punjab, Rajasthan, Uttar Pradesh, Kerala	4
Total				**25**

* Compiled from Table 3.4.

The decline in the prevalence rate for reported as well as for medically treated tuberculosis by NFHS-3 appears possible as a response to efforts made in the control of the disease. This has been confirmed by another independent study[18]. The Central TB Division of the Ministry of Health and Family Welfare has announced a decline of over 12% in the prevalence of infection of tuberculosis in 2007 as compared to the past year. This was based on a survey conducted by TRC (Tuberculosis Research Centre), Chennai. Although, the survey was conducted in Tiruvallur district, 40 kms west of Chennai, the finding was extended to all India on the assumption that if the infection rate fell in one district it must have fallen throughout the country. It was also reported that the transmission of the disease also went down by 6%. The achievement was attributed to DOTS strategy.

Another noteworthy observation is the level of the prevalence rate itself as estimated by various rounds of NFHS and the World Health Organization (WHO). The prevalence rate for all forms of TB in India in 1990 was estimated by WHO in its report for 2006 at 570 per 100,000 persons. It declined to a level of 312 by 2004[19]. The WHO report for 2008 placed the prevalence rates for 1990 and 2006 at 568 and 229 per 100,000 persons. Though two points are insufficient to draw any conclusion on the trend, we may assume a linear decline. The assumption, in the absence of additional data, may be justified on the ground that consistent efforts were made to control TB during the intervening period. This will imply that a decline of 258 points in 14 years or a decline of 269 points in 16 years will mean an average decline of 18 or 17 points per year respectively. This conclusion helps us to estimate the prevalence rate for the disease around the time NFHS-1 and NFHS-2 rounds of the survey were conducted. These estimates may be obtained as 516 or 517 and 426 or 405 respectively, depending upon which WHO report is considered for reference. As stated earlier, NFHS-3 estimated the prevalence

[18]After AIDS, TB cases come down, Teena Thacker, The Indian Express, New Delhi, November 17, 2007.

[19]WHO, op. cit., Table A2.1, p. 214, WHO Report for 2008, Table A3.1.

rate for all forms of TB in 2005–06 at 445 against 299 per 100,000 persons per year.

NFHS estimate of the prevalence rate for reported cases of TB from the first round at 467 per 100,000 persons is 10% lower and that from the second and third rounds at 544 and 445, respectively, is 31% and 49% higher than the comparative estimates derived for corresponding years from WHO data. This contradiction can not be resolved until a third independent source is available. It is interesting to compare the prevalence rate estimated from NFHS-2 for medically treated TB cases with that obtained from WHO data. The former at 445 per 100,000 persons was only about 7% higher than the latter. By contrast the estimate from NFHS-3 for medically treated TB cases at 418 was about 40% higher than that obtained from WHO sources. One possible reason for this difference could be due to the definitions used.

It is further interesting to note that WHO estimated the level of incidence of all forms of TB for 1990, 2004 and 2006 at the same level of incidence of 168 per 100,000 persons per year. The decline in the prevalence rate, despite the continuation of the same incidence rate, may be justified on account of decline in the duration of the disease condition. It may be recalled that incidence rate is inversely related to the period of disease condition and it has been established that DOTS strategy helps in the reduction of the duration of the disease condition thereby reducing the prevalence rate[20]. A study at Tuberculosis Research Centre, Chennai estimated that, in the absence of any control programme, the average duration of disease was about three-and-a-half years. Thus, an incidence rate of 168 per 100,000 persons combined with average duration of disease of 3.5 years will yield a prevalence rate of 588 per 100,000 persons which is very close to 570 given by WHO. The prevalence rate reported by NFHS-1 at 467 combined with incidence rate of 168 given by WHO will yield an average period of disease condition as 2.8 years. Since the estimate of 3.5 years for average duration of

[20]WHO, op. cit., p.20.

disease condition is hard to substantiate to represent the condition at all India level, the estimate derived from NFHS-1 data might be accepted as plausible but on the lower side as it was based on household survey which is liable to suffer from some under-enumeration in view of the fact that people generally like to hide the disease condition particularly in the case of TB. Similar argument, however, might not explain the nature of difference between the estimates from WHO and NFHS-2 and NFHS-3. In this case, it may be noted that NFHS-2 and NFHS-3 asked for medically treated TB cases in addition to the question comparable to that in NFHS-1. This additional effort is likely to increase the prevalence rate.

3.5 URBAN/RURAL DIFFERENTIAL IN PREVALENCE OF TUBERCULOSIS

According to ARTI survey (2000–03) the tuberculosis situation in urban areas was worse than that in rural areas of India. This was shown by estimated prevalence rate of infection of tuberculosis in urban and rural areas at all India level as well as for each of the four zones. At all India level, by pooling the zonal estimates, the annual risk of tuberculosis infection was estimated at 1.5 percent. It was 2.2% for urban areas and 1.3% for rural areas[21]. The estimated ARTI by zone for method-I of the study gives a clear picture of this situation. ARTI in rural areas of north zone at 1.6% was far below that for urban areas at 2.6%. Similar differential was observed in the South, West and East zones with comparative percentages as 0.8, 1.9; 1.5, 2.4 and 1.2, 1.7[22]. This observation is in total disagreement with the general findings that prevalence and incidence of tuberculosis are negatively related to the state of socio-economic development. According to this, the values of ARTI in the urban

[21]VK Chadha, P Kumar, PS Jagannatha et al, Average risk of tuberculosis infection in India, Int J Tuberc Lung Dis 2005; 9 (1): 116–118.

[22]Annual Risk of Tuberculosis Infection in Different Zones of India, A National Sample Survey, 2000–2003 by VK Chadha, SP Agarwal, LS Chauhan given in Tuberculosis Control in India, SP Agarwal and LS Chauhan, Directorate General of Health Service, Ministry of Health and Family Welfare, New Delhi, 2005.

areas should have been lower than that in the rural areas. Prevalence of tuberculosis as revealed by national level household survey data in India as contained in NFHS Reports described below has shown that urban areas were generally better than rural areas. A similar finding is also reported for China for the year 2003, where prevalence rates of tuberculosis were negatively related to the level of socio-economic development. For example, the rate per 100,000 persons per year for urban areas increased from 37 to 150 with decreasing level of socio-economic development in three categories for urban areas. Similar observation was noted for rural areas where the rate increased from 81 to 223 as the level of development decreased from level I to level IV[23].

NFHS survey results relating to prevalence of TB in urban and rural areas of India appear to be at variance from the findings of ARTI survey[24]. The available data from the household survey provide the urban-rural segregation for the prevalence rate for all forms of tuberculosis in three rounds of the survey and that for medically treated tuberculosis for the 2nd and 3rd rounds at all India level. The rates for 1998–99 refer to the situation closer to the time period of the ARTI survey conducted during 2000–03. NFHS data shows that TB, all forms as well as medically treated, was more prevalent in rural than in urban areas in the country. For example, the reported prevalence rate of tuberculosis in rural areas was at least 50% higher than that in urban areas. It may be obtained from Table 3.6 that the rural/urban differential measured by percentage of rural to urban rate varied from 49% for 1992–93 to 57% for 2005–06, with 54% for 1998–99. Similar differential stood for even the medically treated tuberculosis where it stood at 55% and 53% for 1998–99 and 2005–06 respectively.

Differential similar to that noted above may be seen for state level prevalence of tuberculosis in rural and urban areas. Twenty of the 25 states for which data were available for

---

[23]*M Zhongwci Zhao:* Income Inequality, unequal Health Census Access and Marketing in China, Population and Development Review, Vol, 32 (3), September 2006 P. 471.

[24]Refer to Table 3.6 of this chapter.

Table 3.6: Number of persons per 100,000 household population (prevalence rate) suffering from tuberculosis by area of residence, India, 1992–93, 1998–99 and 2005–06 (NFHS data)

Survey period	*Area of residence*		
	Rural	**Urban**	**Total**
All forms of tuberculosis			
1992–93	512	344	467
1998–99	600	390	544
2005–06	502	319	445
Medically treated tuberculosis			
1998–99	476	307	432
2005–06	469	307	418

1998–99 round of NFHS, prevalence rates for reported cases of tuberculosis were lower in urban than in rural areas. Exceptions were noted in Delhi in the north, Mizoram, Nagaland and Tripura in the northeast and Maharashtra in the west. Of these exceptions only Maharashtra is a large state. A somewhat similar differential may be noted for medically treated TB as well. In the latter case six of the 25 states showed higher rate of prevalence for tuberculosis in urban than in rural areas. These were Delhi in the north, Manipur, Mizoram and Nagaland in the northeast and Goa and Maharashtra in the west. The details are given in Table 3.7. The above contradiction even in the case of medically treated tuberculosis which presumably, because of its linkage with medical certification, reflects the truth, is hard to justify. In the absence of a third reliable source, the contradiction of the findings of ARTI survey and household surveys is hard to reconcile. Since ARTI data were based on medical testing of children below the age of ten years and NFHS data were collected through interviewing the head or any other knowledgeable adult in the household, it is difficult to draw a definite conclusion about the differential. It is quite possible, that both of these sources are telling some sort of truth about the prevalence of the disease in the population. It appears that the occurrence of slums in urban areas (where living conditions might be worse than that in rural areas because of deterioration in the quality of life in urban

Table 3.7: Number of persons per 100,000 household population suffering from tuberculosis by state and residence, India, 1998–99

	All reported cases			*Medically treated tuberculosis*		
	Total	**Urban**	**Rural**	**Urban**	**Rural**	**Total**
India	544	390	600	307	476	432
North						
Delhi	511	548	92	483	92	451
Haryana	358	305	379	284	327	314
Himachal Pradesh	259	200	265	177	240	234
Jammu & Kashmir	428	320	455	320	455	428
Punjab	207	200	210	164	210	197
Rajasthan	397	329	420	290	358	342
Central						
Madhya Pradesh	602	405	669	326	587	520
Uttar Pradesh	551	490	566	347	444	424
East						
Bihar	989	629	1035	558	868	833
Orissa	833	819	835	652	714	707
West Bengal	492	357	537	170	330	290
Northeast						
Arunachal Pradesh	1270	1055	1302	792	1164	1115
Assam	710	583	721	345	358	357
Manipur	1107	1086	1118	1086	988	1020
Meghalaya	1459	580	1679	506	683	648
Mizoram	1063	1096	1027	907	708	813
Nagaland	1654	1723	1637	1546	961	1078
Tripura	1002	1151	980	128	742	662
West						
Goa	466	445	480	329	304	314
Gujarat	438	279	550	242	438	357
Maharashtra	282	342	236	282	191	230
South						
Andhra Pradesh	592	299	695	199	532	446
Karnataka	269	216	297	190	237	221
Kerala	526	348	581	301	434	403
Tamil Nadu	479	431	505	366	455	424

Source: Table 6.8, NF HS-2.

areas) induces higher prevalence of TB in such areas as observed by the ARTI survey. On the other hand, poverty in rural areas, a factor positively linked with TB, may be responsible for higher prevalence of TB in rural areas as observed by the NFHS surveys. Another factor which could play an important role in this odd differential which needs investigation is inflation of TB cases in urban areas arising out of lack of medical facilities in rural areas forcing the rural population to urban centres for treatment. If an independent research confirms the findings of the ARTI survey as reflecting the truth about prevalence of tuberculosis in the country then it will raise a question on the planning process which encourages urbanization but at the same time it induces spread of tuberculosis. Hopefully future research will be able to shed light on this important aspect and assist in developing suitable strategies for controlling tuberculosis.

3.6 PREVALENCE OF TUBERCULOSIS BY AGE, GENDER AND PLACE OF RESIDENCE

National Family Health Survey provides data on prevalence rate of tuberculosis by age and gender as well as by rural/urban residence. The data for all India are summarized in Table 3.8. The distribution of prevalence rate by age from the three rounds of the survey is directly comparable for only the age group 15–59 years. Detailed distribution available from the first round for ages below 15 and above 60 years have been merged together in the subsequent rounds. Irrespective of the level of the rate, it may be noted that, the prevalence of TB is very much age dependent, both for all reported as well as medically treated tuberculosis. The prevalence increases with advancing age. Senior citizens aged 60 + years were twice as likely to have TB as those in the economically active age group (15–59 years). This was true for reported as well as for medically treated cases. The pattern is consistently shown for various rounds of the NFHS survey. The prevalence was substantially lower for children aged less than 15 years and was almost at one-fourth level as that for economically active persons. It appears, that the rates for smaller age divisions for children or for aged persons were very close as revealed by data for 1992–93 and this might have prompted the merger of the age groups in the subsequent rounds. The overall reduction in the prevalence rate is reflected in lowering of rates for each of the age groups considered. We may take the liberty of putting the prevalence rate of tuberculosis at about 100, 500 and 1000 per 100,000 persons for age groups less than 15, 15–59 and 60 + years respectively.

The association between gender and prevalence of tuberculosis is not that clear as that by age. For example, data for 1st and 2nd rounds of NFHS showed that males were more likely to have TB than females. By contrast the reverse is demonstrated by data for the 3rd round of the survey. While the prevalence rate for males in 1992–93 and 1998–99 was respectively 54% and 36% higher than the rate for females, in 2005–06 it was 40% lower. The medically treated tuberculosis showed similar differential.

The pattern of overall differential was exhibited by each of the urban and rural areas separately, though with different magnitude. For example, the reported level of prevalence of tuberculosis for senior citizens in rural areas at 1448 per 100,000 persons in 1998–99 was about 87% higher than that for economically productive persons compared with 168% for urban areas. Data for 2005–06 showed similar differential for rural areas with actual rates lower than those for 1998–99 but the differential for the urban areas was only 109% higher than that for urban areas. Overall, a rural male aged 60 + years was the most vulnerable group to contact TB. Details are summarized in Table 3.8.

New smear-positive case notification rates by age and gender for India in 2004 given by WHO[25] also show the age and gender dependence of the disease as that shown by NFHS data with the exception that those in the 65 + age group in WHO data had lower notification rate than the ages below that. Despite the limitations of data considered here, the consistency of trend shows clearly that TB is quite common among males in the economically productive age segment. Such a pattern is a matter of concern as most of these patients are also the bread-winners for the family.

[25]WHO, op. cit., Table A.2.9, p. 222.

Table 3.8: Number of persons per 100,000 household population suffering from tuberculosis according to age, gender and residence, India, 1992–93, 1998–99 and 2005–06

	Year of survey								
	1992-93			*1998-99*			*2005-06*		
	Urban	**Rural**	**Total**	**Urban**	**Rural**	**Total**	**Urban**	**Rural**	**Total**
Age	**Reported cases of tuberculosis (includes medically treated cases)**								
0–4	140	81	95	Rates merged with the next age group					
5–14	181	117	132	144	155	153	98	115	110
15–59	368	617	546	426	776	675	367	653	555
60–69	998	1812	1623	1141	1448	1374	768	1180	1066
70+	1033	1731	1569	Rates merged with the previous age group					
Gender									
Male	397	625	564	446	690	624	247	371	334
Female	286	393	365	330	507	460	385	634	554
Total	344	512	467	390	600	544	319	502	445
Age	**Medically treated tuberculosis**								
0–14	na	na	na	106	106	106	98	114	110
15–59	na	na	na	338	630	545	354	605	519
60+	na	na	na	913	1141	1086	727	1102	998
Gender									
Male	na	na	na	350	558	502	246	337	309
Female	na	na	na	262	391	357	364	602	526
Total	na	na	na	307	476	432	307	469	418

Source: Table 8.1, NFHS-1; Table 6.7, NFHS-2 and Table 13.1.1, NFHS-3.

The rise in the infection/prevalence rate for tuberculosis with increase in age is also exhibited in Table 3.9.

Table 3.9: Infection rate for tuberculosis in India

Age group (Yrs)	*Infected (%)*
0–4	1.0
5–9	6.4
10–14	15.4
15–24	31.9
25–34	47.3
35–44	54.8
45–54	60.7
55 and above	62.1
Total	**30.4**

http://www.medindia.net/health_statistics/diseases/tb.asp

3.7 SOME RELATED ASPECTS OF PREVALENCE OF TB

Drug-resistant TB in India

MDR TB in India and the World[26]

The community-based drug resistance surveillance (DRS) conducted in Indian states of Gujarat and Maharashtra showed that the incidence of MDR-TB was estimated to be about three percent among the new cases. According to RNTCP, the MDR-TB levels in India are about three percent in new cases and 12–17 percent in re-treatment cases. However, a 2004 WHO Global TB Control Study in India estimated the level of MDR-TB in the country at 4.1 percent of the total estimated number of cases of new and previously treated TB cases.

In addition to surveys in Gujarat and Maharashtra, it was noted that incidence of MRD-TB among those patients who came for re-treatment was as high as 12 to 17 percent. This estimate could be on the lower side. This is because tests to ascertain whether a patient suffered from the drug resistant TB had to be conducted only in accredited labs where it takes 15 days for the results. The number of such labs in the country was only six at the time. Plan was to develop ten more centers in next two years.

[26]Savita Verma, Mail Today, New Delhi, December 15, 2007.

Providing treatment for MDR-TB requires training of health care workers to see how patients were responding to treatment. Besides, patients also needed daily injections for six months and sputum testing every month. Presently about 60,000 patients in India may be in need of treatment for MDR-TB. This may be on lower side. The cost per patient works out to be Rs 1,20,000. In contrast, the cost of treating drug susceptible TB is just Rs. 500 to Rs. 600 per patient and patients can get cured in six to eight months.

Globally, in terms of absolute number, WHO estimated that there were over 4,00,000 cases of MDR-TB every year, with estimated deaths of over 1,00,000. China, India and the Russian Federation contributed to a majority of this case burden, with India itself contributing 80,000 cases every year. The figures have gone up somewhat lately. WHO's global report on drug resistant TB for 2008 estimated that about 440,000 people globally got infected with MDR TB in 2008 while 150,000 died of it. Progress in the treatment was slow in most countries. Worldwide, of those patients receiving treatment, 60% were cured. Diagnosis of MDR TB was a matter of concern as only an estimated 7% of all such cases were detected. Therefore, WHO rightly pointed to the fact that there was an urgent need to expand and accelerate diagnosis capabilities in countries and have technology that could diagnose MDR TB in two days rather than traditional methods that could take up to four months.

XDR-TB in India and the World

The world's most untreatable form of tuberculosis, extreme drug-resistant TB (XDR-TB), has been detected in India and could account for about 8% of those who suffer from the strain of the disease. National TB Control Programme has no official data on the prevalence of XDR-TB in India. The Union Health Ministry had feared that detection of strain was a matter of time. The concern was that it was nearly impossible to determine prevalence of XDR-TB in India[27].

In India where TB prevalence is quite wide spread and that patients often do not complete recommended treatment, the

[27]Times of India, May 23, 2007.

discovery of XDR-TB is not surprising. Two studies have, however, lately revealed disturbing findings about infection of extensively drug-resistant tuberculosis (XDR-TB) among India's HIV patients[28]. A study conducted by AIIMS's clinical microbiology department found that over 33% of those enrolled for the study, with both HIV and TB, were suffering from XDR-TB. Further, all the patients with XDR-TB died within three months of diagnosis. Fifty-four AIDS patients suspected of having HIV-tuberculosis co-infection were investigated in 2006 for the prevalence of XDR-TB. Out of them, TB was isolated from 24 (44.4%). Twelve (50%) of these had resistance to first-line drugs, whereas four (33.33%) were also resistant to second-line drugs. This was the first large scale study done in India with subjects being co-infected with HIV and TB. It was also the first time that XDR-TB was found to infect HIV patients in India.

The above study, though, appeared months after researchers from Hinduja National Hospital in Mumbai had detected XDR-TB in 8% of all TB patients. The team had examined 3,904 lab samples and found 1,274 were positive for TB of these, 32% were multiple drug resistance (MDR-TB), of which 8% were XDR-TB cases. Mortality rate of XDR-TB patients in the study was as high as 42%. The worrying observation was that majority of patients in the study with XDR-TB were from a younger age group, their average age being 30 years All XDR-TB cases were in-patients with pulmonary tuberculosis which can spread by coughing, sneezing, laughing or even singing. The AIIMS and Hinduja figures could not be extrapolated because these were tertiary referral hospitals getting the worst patients. Also, the AIIMS sample size is too small. TB is the single largest killer of AIDS patients in India. NACO reveals that over 60% of all AIDS patients contract and ultimately die of TB.

Globally XDR-TB strain has been detected in 37 countries. The true scale of XDR-TB, however, is unknown as many countries lack the necessary equipment and capacity to accurately diagnose it. WHO estimated that, there were around

[28]Drug-resistant TB infecting HIV+ in India, Times of India, New Delhi, December 26, 2007.

40,000 cases per year. As of June 2008, 49 countries had confirmed cases of XDR-TB.

At least 50 percent of those who contract this strain of Tuberculosis eventually die of it. To stop the spread sometimes extreme degree of control is imposed on the infected people. A ray of hope has however come from a Russian trial on 608 MDR-TB patients, 4.8% of whom had XDR-TB[29]. Russian trial used aggressive therapy, with each patient given at least five drugs he was susceptible to. The result showed that 48% of XDR-TB patients responded favourably.

The replication of Russian trial for treating XDR-TB in India done at Hinduja hospital gave a survival rate of 40% for XDR-TB patients. India may find it hard to replicate Russian experiment because it is expensive and needs well-structured TB programmes. Our government labs and programmes have no such set-ups and drugs are not provided except in some pilot projects. It has not helped either to have poor patients with little knowledge, poor resistance and little government aid. Besides, there are no more drugs in TB which can combat the extreme resistance among XDR-TB patients.

3.8 TUBERCULOSIS AS A CAUSE OF DEATH IN INDIA

Medical Certification of Causes of Death (MCCD) introduced in the 1960s under Section 10 of the Registration of Births and Deaths Act, 1969 in almost all the States/Union Territories of India operated at different levels of efficiency across the states in terms of coverage, reporting and quality of data. Owing to these limitations, the cause specific mortality flowing from MCCD was far from satisfactory. To mitigate the situation the 'Survey of Causes of Death' initiated in rural areas was merged with the Sample Registration System (SRS) from 1999, thus encompassing both rural and urban areas. Since then, a system of Verbal Autopsy under the domain of SRS has been in operation.

In order to effect improvement in the system, the Office of the Registrar General, India (ORGI) in collaboration with the Centre for Global Health Research (CGHR), University of Toronto has been trying to establish a reliable system to

[29]Sunday Times of India, New Delhi, August 31, 2008.

measure the status of causes-specific deaths in the country. Thus, the Special Survey of Deaths (SSD), 2001–03, under the domain of Sample Registration System (SRS) covered over 6,645 small areas (sample units) in all the States and Union Territories. The causes of death have been determined using an advanced form of Verbal Autopsy - "RHIME" or Representative, Re-sampled, Routine Household Interview of Mortality - with Medical Evaluation method. A random sample of about 5-10% of the units was resurveyed by an independent team to ensure the quality of fieldwork, completeness and accuracy. The assignment of causes of death was done through a medical evaluation by two independent trained physicians who had examined the field reports using a web-based system developed specifically for the study. The cases resulting into continuing disagreements were referred to a third physician to adjudicate the final ICD-10 code. The SSD 2004–05 covered deaths from 2001–03 in SRS.

The mortality picture revealed, according to the Report, has to be interpreted carefully as the chance of misclassification of causes is not completely ruled out. Despite this limitation, the Report is hopeful that the study brings out findings which should definitely help enrich understanding of the mortality situation and challenges thereof in the country. We concentrate here only on deaths caused by TB.

Share of Overall Death due to TB

Spatial Units

The published Report[30], based on the distribution of 113,692 deaths (62,653 male and 51,039 female) presents the status of ten leading causes of death in India. Here we will take only the deaths caused by TB. However, it may be observed that overall the top ten leading causes of death are cardiovascular disease (19%), followed by respiratory diseases (9%), diarrhoeal diseases (8%), perinatal conditions (6.3%), respiratory infections such as acute pneumonia (6.2%), tuberculosis (6%), malignant and other

[30]Report on Causes of Death in India 2001–03, Office of Registrar General, Ministry of Home Affairs, Government of India, New Delhi in collaboration with Center for Global Health Research, St. Michael's Hospital, University of Toronto, Canada.

neoplasms (5.7%), senility (5.1%), unintentional injuries (4.9%), and symptoms, signs and ill-defined conditions (4.8%).

The data are also given for EAG states[31] and Assam as one group and other states as another.

As noted above TB was the 6th ranked cause of death in the country accounting for 6.0 per cent of all deaths, more male than female deaths (7.1% and 4.7% respectively). EAG and Assam accounted for higher percentage of deaths due to TB than other states. It is surprising that TB, despite accounting for lower share of deaths in urban areas (5.3%), was the fourth ranked cause of death as against sixth ranked in rural areas (6.1%). The ranking and the corresponding percentage of all deaths accounted for by TB according to spatial group and gender is given in Table 3.10.

Table 3.10: Rank and percentage of deaths caused by TB among all deaths (SSD data), by spatial group and gender, India, 2001–03

	Gender			
Rank	*Male*	*Female*	*Persons*	*Spatial group*
6th	7.1	4.7	6.0	India
6th	8.1	5.2	6.7	EAG states and Assam
6th	6.3	4.1	5.3	Other states
6th	7.3	4.7	6.1	Rural
4th	5.9	4.5	5.3	Urban

By Regions

Share of deaths due to TB varied within a narrow range from 5.1% in the south to a high of 7.2% in the central region. The wide difference between percentages for central and eastern regions at 7.2% and 5.4% is somewhat surprising as the two are comprised of states in the neighbouring areas. The central region comprised of Madhya Pradesh, Chhattisgarh, Rajasthan and Uttar Pradesh while eastern region included Bihar, Jharkhand, Orissa and West Bengal. Table 3.11 presents the detailed rankings and the corresponding share of death due to TB among all deaths.

[31]EAG (Empowered Action Group) includes states such as Bihar, Jharkhand, Madhya Pradesh, Chhattisgarh, Orissa, Rajasthan, Uttar Pradesh and Uttarakhand.

Table 3.11: Rank and percentage of deaths caused by TB among all deaths (SSD data), by region and gender, India, 2001–03

Rank	*Gender*			*Region*
	Male	*Female*	*Persons*	
6th	7.1	4.7	6.0	India
7th	6.0	4.1	5.2	North
6th	7.3	5.4	6.5	North-East
7th	6.5	4.2	5.4	East
6th	8.6	5.7	7.2	Central
5th	7.7	4.3	6.2	West
7th	6.0	4.0	5.1	South

By Age and Gender

The available data for ten leading causes of death in India by age show that TB appears as one of the top ten causes of death only in the age group 5–14 years at rank 9th in the EAG states and Assam. Thereafter TB appears as one of the top ten causes of death in all the subsequent age groups irrespective of the spatial unit considered as shown in Table 3.12.

Deaths due to TB rank higher in the more productive age groups. The most economically productive age range of 25–69 years recorded the deaths due to TB at rank three, with variation from rank 2 to 4 depending upon the spatial unit. The next age group is 15–24 years where it occupies 5th rank, varying between 4th and 7th. In age group 70+, TB as a cause of death comes only at 8th rank, and varies between 5th and 9th. The age group 15–24 is dominated by deaths caused by violent events which occupy top four ranks (intentional self-harm (16%), unintentional injuries: other (12%), symptoms signs and ill-defined conditions (7%), Motor vehicle accidents (7%). The top two causes of death in age group 25–69 are cardiovascular diseases (25%), and respiratory diseases (namely chronic obstructive pulmonary disease (COPD, asthma, and other respiratory disease) (10.2%). Table 3.12 gives the rank and percentage of deaths among all deaths caused by TB according to broad age group and gender for specified spatial units.

Table 3.12: Rank and percentage of deaths among all deaths caused by TB (SSD data), according to broad age group and gender for specified spatial units, India, 2001–03

						Age group in years						
	15–24				*25–69*				*70+*			
												Spatial group
		Gender		*Rank*		*Gender*		*Rank*		*Gender*		
	M	*F*	*P*		*M*	*F*	*P*		*M*	*F*	*P*	
5th	6.0	7.5	6.8	3rd	11.4	8.3	10.1	8th	4.5	2.6	3.6	India
4th	8.9	9.0	9.0	2nd	14.8	10.1	12.8	5th	5.0	3.3	4.2	EAG states and Assam
7th	3.7	5.9	4.8	4th	9.1	6.9	8.3	9th	4.1	2.1	3.0	Other states
6th	6.0	7.2	6.6	3rd	12.2	8.6	10.7	7th	4.7	2.6	3.7	Rural
5th	6.4	10.0	8.1	3rd	8.2	6.9	7.7	9th	3.5	2.4	2.9	Urban

Note: M = Male, F = Female, P = Person

Appendix Table 3.1: Estimated epidemiological burden of TB, 2007

		Number in 000s and Rates per 1,00,000 population per year										
Country/Region		*Incidence*				*Prevalence*		*Mortality*				
		All forms		*Smear +*		*All forms*		*HIV –*		*HIV +*		*HIV prev.in incident TB cases %*
High-burden countries (HBCs)	*Rank*	*Number*	*Rate*	*Number*	*Rate*	*Number*	*Rate*	*Number*	*Rate*	*Number*	*Rate*	
India	1	1962	168	873	75	3305	283	302	26	30	2.5	5.3
HBCs Neighbouring countries												
China	2	1306	98	585	44	2582	194	194	15	6.8	0.5	1.9
Bangladesh	6	353	223	159	100	614	387	70	44	0.4	0.3	0.3
Pakistan	8	297	181	133	81	365	223	46	28	1.4	0.9	2.1
Other HBCs												
Indonesia	3	528	228	236	102	566	244	86	37	5.4	2.4	3
Nigeria	4	460	311	195	131	772	521	79	53	59	40	27
South Africa	5	461	948	174	358	336	692	18	38	94	193	73
Ethiopia	7	314	378	135	163	481	579	53	64	23	28	19
Philippines	9	255	290	115	130	440	500	36	41	0.3	0.3	0.3
DR Congo	10	245	392	109	174	417	666	45	72	6	10	5.9

Contd...

Appendix Table 3.1: Estimated epidemiological burden of TB, 2007 (*Contd...*)

Number in 000s and Rates per 1,00,000 population per year												
Country/Region		*Incidence*				*Prevalence*		*Mortality*				
		All forms		*Smear +*		*All forms*		*HIV –*		*HIV +*		*HIV prev.in incident TB cases %*
High-burden countries (HBCs)	*Rank*	*Number*	*Rate*	*Number*	*Rate*	*Number*	*Rate*	*Number*	*Rate*	*Number*	*Rate*	
Russian	11	157	110	68	48	164	115	20	14	5.1	3.6	16
Viet Nam	12	150	171	66	76	192	220	18	20	3.1	3.5	8.1
Kenya	13	132	353	53	142	120	319	10	26	15	39	48
Brazil	14	92	48	49	26	114	60	5.9	3.1	2.5	1.3	14
UR Tanzania	15	120	297	49	120	136	337	12	29	20	49	47
Uganda	16	102	330	42	136	132	426	13	41	16	52	39
Zimbabwe	17	104	782	40	298	95	714	6.9	52	28	213	69
Thailand	18	91	142	39	62	123	192	10	15	3.9	6	17
Mozambique	19	92	431	37	174	108	504	10	45	17	82	47
Myanmar	20	83	171	37	75	79	162	5.4	11	0.9	1.9	11
Combodia	21	72	495	32	219	96	664	11	77	1.8	13	7.8
Afghanistan	22	46	168	21	76	65	238	8.2	30	0	0	0
HBCs		**7423**	**177**	**3245**	**77**	**11301**	**269**	**1058**	**25**	**339**	**8.1**	**14**

Contd...

Appendix Table 3.1: Estimated epidemiological burden of TB, 2007 (*Contd...*)

Number in 000s and Rates per 1,00,000 population per year											
Country/Region	*Incidence*				*Prevalence*		*Mortality*				
	All forms		*Smear +*		*All forms*		*HIV –*		*HIV +*		*HIV prev.in incident TB cases %*
High-burden countries (HBCs)	*Number*	*Rate*	*Number*	*Rate*	*Number*	*Rate*	*Number*	*Rate*	*Number*	*Rate*	
Regions											
AFR	2879	363	1188	150	3766	475	357	45	378	48	38
AMR	295	32	157	17	348	38	33	3.6	7.9	0.9	11
EMR	583	105	259	47	772	139	97	17	7.7	1.4	3.5
EUR	432	49	190	21	456	51	56	6.3	8.1	0.9	9.8
SEAR	3165	181	1410	81	4881	280	497	28	40	2.3	4.6
WPR	1919	108	859	48	3500	197	276	16	15	0.8	2.7
Global	**9273**	**139**	**4062**	**61**	**13723**	**206**	**1316**	**20**	**456**	**6.8**	**15**

Incidence and prevalence estimates include TB in people with HIV Prevalence of HIV incident TB cases of all ages.

Source: WHO: Global Tuberculosis Control 2009: Epidemiology, Strategy, Financing. WHO Report 2009, Geneva, World Health Organization (Table 1.2).

Note:
AFR = WHO Africa Region.
AMR = WHO Region of the Americas.
EMR = WHO Eastern Mediterranean Region.
EUR = WHO European Region.
SEAR = WHO South-East Asia Region.
WPR = WHO Western Pacific Region.

4

Management and Control

"India has made remarkable progress in expanding the internationally recommended DOTS Strategy to 97% of the country. The challenge is to sustain good quality services, widen the reach through involvement of wider network of healthcare providers, and deal with newer challenges posed by TB-HIV Co-infection and drug resistance."

Dr. SJ Habayeb
WHO Representative to India

4.1 INTRODUCTION

In view of the huge economic, social and health etc., costs and increasing burden, tuberculosis has become a matter of prime concern to national governments in many countries and the international bodies. At the latter level the World Health Organization (WHO) has been the primary agent for prevention, control and management of the disease. From the global standpoint, in spite of reduction in many parts, tuberculosis continues to be a major public health problem. According to WHO Expert Committee Report of 1959, "With the encouraging progress made in the control of malaria, tuberculosis now is the most important specific communicable disease in the world as a whole and its control should receive priority and emphasis both by WHO and the governments". This observation made almost half a century ago is still valid with somewhat similar intensity. The problem is most serious in the developing countries of Asia, Africa and South America, where the disease is particularly damaging because of the chronic illness and the mortality to which it gives rise in the productive adults section of the population. This chapter is an attempt to describe efforts made by WHO and Indian system in the area of prevention, control and management of tuberculosis.

In order to raise all around awareness about the disease, its prevention, control, management etc., March 24 each year is commemorated as World Tuberculosis Day across the globe. This symbolizes the date in 1882 when Robert Koch announced the discovery of mycobacterium tuberculosis, the causative bacterium of TB, at Berlin in Germany. At that time, it was considered a dreaded disease killing millions, as it was causing death of one out of every seven people, not only in Europe but other continents as well.

4.2 GLOBAL ACTIONS BY WHO[1]

WHO, as world leader in health management and control, has been assessing the status of the TB epidemic and progress in control of the disease every year since 1997. This assessment has included estimates of TB incidence, prevalence and mortality (from 1990 onwards); analysis of case notifications (from 1995) and treatment outcomes (from 1994) in around 200 (of 212) countries and territories. In addition, the organization has been carrying out the analysis of progress towards the global targets for case detection and treatment success which were established by the World Health Assembly (WHA) in 1991. Since 2006, WHO has also assessed progress towards achieving the impact targets related to incidence, prevalence and mortality that have been set for 2015 within the framework of the millennium development goals (MDGs) and by the Stop TB Partnership. The global targets and indicators for TB control were developed within the framework of the MDGs as well as

[1]Most of the presentation in this section is based on World Health Organization's Report "Global Tuberculosis" Control 2009: Epidemiology, Strategy, Financing.

by the Stop TB Partnership and the World Health Assembly. These are presented in Box 1[2].

Box 1: Goals, targets and indicators for TB control

Health in the Millennium Development Goals

Goal 6: Combat HIV/AIDS, malaria and other diseases.

Target 6c: Halt and begin to reverse the incidence of malaria and other major diseases.

Indicator 6.9: Incidence, prevalence and death rates associated with TB

Indicator 6.10: Proportion of TB cases detected and cured under DOTS

Stop TB Partnership Targets

By 2005: At least 70% of people with sputum smear-positive TB will be diagnosed (i.e. under the DOTS strategy), and at least 85% successfully treated. The targets of a case detection rate of at least 70% and a treatment success rate of at least 85% were first set by the World Health Assembly of WHO in 1991.

By 2015: The global burden of TB (per capita prevalence and death rates) will be reduced by 50% relative to 1990 levels.

By 2050: The global incidence of active TB will be less than case detection rate of at least 70% and 1 case per million population per year.

Since the purpose of international and national efforts is to control TB, it is necessary to devise techniques for accurate and reliable assessment of incidence, prevalence and mortality rates. Demonstrating whether or not they are achieved is of major importance for individual countries, the United Nations, WHO and the Stop TB Partnership, and a variety of technical, financial and development agencies. To meet this requirement, WHO Global Task Force on TB Impact Measurement developed guidelines. These are used to obtain the estimates of incidence, prevalence and mortality rates of TB and their trends based on the best available data and analytical methods, both of which were reviewed and endorsed by a group of experts in mid-2008. These policy guidelines are given in Box 2[3]. As and when better surveillance systems, additional survey data, more in-depth analysis of existing surveillance and programmatic data and further refinement of analytical methods become available,

[2]Ibid Table 1.1.

[3]Ibid Table 1.3.

these estimates could be improved in the period up to 2015 and beyond.

Box 2: WHO policy package for measuring rates of TB incidence, prevalence and mortality, 2008–2015 and beyond

General

1. Improve surveillance systems to include all (or almost all) incident cases in TB case notification data and to account for all (or almost all) TB deaths in vital registration systems.
2. Strengthen national capacity to monitor and evaluate the TB epidemic and to measure progress in TB control.
3. Review and update periodically the data, assumptions and analytical methods used to produce WHO estimates of TB incidence, prevalence and mortality rates.
4. Report by Task Force on whether 2015 MDG and Stop TB Partnership targets are achieved (or not), shortly after 2015.

Measuring TB incidence rates

5. Analyse periodically the reliability and coverage of case notification data using a standard framework, in order to estimate the total number of incident TB cases and trends in incidence rates.
6. Certify and/or validate TB notification data for countries where analyses using the standard framework show that TB notification data are a close proxy (direct measure) of TB incidence.
7. Cross-validate estimates of TB incidence using TB mortality data from vital registration systems.

Measuring TB prevalence rates

8. Survey the prevalence of TB disease in 21 global focus countries according to WHO guidelines and Task Force recommendations.
9. Produce indirect estimates of TB prevalence based on estimates of TB incidence and the duration of TB disease for countries where surveys of the prevalence of TB disease are not implemented.

Measuring TB mortality rates

10. Develop national vital registration systems to reliably record all TB deaths.
11. Initiate sample vital registration where national vital registration systems are not yet available.
12. Produce indirect estimates of TB mortality using estimates of TB incidence and case fatality rates for countries without reliable national or sample vital registration systems.

Evaluating the impact of TB control

13. Conduct studies periodically to evaluate the impact of control on rates of TB incidence, prevalence and mortality.

Stop TB Strategy

The Stop TB Strategy launched by WHO in 2006 is designed to achieve the targets set for 2015 (Box 1). It has six major components: (i) DOTS expansion and enhancement; (ii) addressing TB/HIV, MDR-TB and other challenges; (iii) contributing to health system strengthening; (iv) engaging all care providers; (v) empowering patients and communities; and (vi) enabling and promoting research. Details are given in Box 3[4]. Technical elements of the DOTS strategy are given in Box 4[5].

Box 3: Components of the Stop TB strategy

1. **Pursue high-quality DOTS expansion and enhancement**
   a. Secure political commitment, with adequate and sustained financing.
   b. Ensure early case detection, and diagnosis through quality-assured bacteriology.
   c. Provide standardized treatment with supervision, and patient support.
   d. Ensure effective drug supply and management.
   e. Monitor and evaluate performance and impact.
2. **Address TB-HIV, MDR-TB, and the needs of poor and vulnerable populations**
   a. Scale up collaborative TB/HIV activities.
   b. Scale up prevention and management of multidrug-resistant TB (MDR-TB).
   c. Address the needs of TB contacts, and of poor and vulnerable populations, including women, children, prisoners, refugees, migrants and ethnic minorities.
3. **Contribute to health system strengthening based on primary health care**
   a. Help improve health policies, human resource development, financing, supplies, service delivery and information.
   b. Strengthen infection control in health services, other congregate settings and households.
   c. Upgrade laboratory networks, and implement the Practical Approach to Lung Health (PAL).

[4]Ibid Table 2.1.
[5]Ibid Table 2.2.

   d. Adapt successful approaches from other fields and sectors, and foster action on the social determinants of health.

4. **Engage all care providers**
   a. Involve all public, voluntary, corporate and private providers through Public-Private Mix (PPM) approaches.
   b. Promote use of the International Standards for TB Care (ISTC).
5. **Empower people with TB, and communities through partnership**
   a. Pursue advocacy, communication and social mobilization.
   b. Foster community participation in TB care.
   c. Promote use of the Patient's Charter for TB Care.
6. **Enable and promote research**
   a. Conduct programme-based operational research, and introduce new tools into practice.
   b. Advocate for and participate in research to develop new diagnostics, drugs and vaccines.

Box 4: Technical elements of the DOTS strategy

Case detection through quality–assured bacteriology

Sputum smear microscopy should be used to detect cases among symptomatic patients self-reporting to health services. Sputum culture is also used for diagnosis in some countries, but direct sputum smear microscopy should still be performed for all suspected cases.

Standardized treatment with supervision and patient support

Use standardized short-course chemotherapy using regimens of 6–8 months for at least all confirmed smear-positive cases. Good case management includes directly observed treatment (DOT) during the intensive phase for all new smear-positive cases, during the continuation phase of regimens containing rifampicin and during the entirety of a re-treatment regimen. In countries that have consistently documented high rates of treatment success, DOT may be reserved for a subset of patients, as long as cohort analysis of treatment results is provided to document the outcome of all cases.

An effective drug supply and management system

Establish and maintain a system to supply all essential anti-TB drugs and Ensure no interruption in their availability.

Monitoring and evaluation system, and impact measurement

Establish and maintain a standardized recording and reporting system, allowing assessment of treatment results.

In order to facilitate the development of policy to guide the implementation of new diagnostic tools, WHO has established a structured process for evaluating and translating research findings into policy and practice (the latest WHO policy on TB diagnosis is summarized in Box 5)[6]. Ongoing monitoring will be used to assess the uptake of these tools and their impact on diagnosis and treatment outcomes. In most resource-constrained countries, uptake of new tools requires considerable strengthening of laboratory infrastructure, deployment of additional human resources and funding for the purchase of new technologies.

Box 5: Recent WHO policy changes in diagnosis of TB

1. WHO policy on smear microscopy and case detection

With the prerequisite of a functional external microscopy quality assurance (EQA) system, with blinded rechecking, the new definition of a smear-positive TB case is "a patient with one or more initial sputum smear examinations positive for acid fast bacilli (AFB)". Further information including evidence for this policy can be found at: http://www.who.int/tb/dots/laboratory/policy/en/index1.html

2. WHO policy on the Use of liquid medium for culture and drug susceptibility testing (DST) in middle-income and low-income countries.

WHO recommends the use of commercial liquid systems (the standard of care for TB diagnosis and patient management in developed countries) for culture and DST in middle-income and low-income countries, within the context of national laboratory strengthening plans and using a phased approach to implementation at the country level. Further information including prerequisites for the phased introduction of this technology can be found at: http://www.who.int/tb/dots/laboratory/policy/en/index3 html

3. WHO policy on the use of molecular line probe assays

WHO recommends the use of molecular line probe assays for the rapid detection of MDR-TB cases, within the context of national laboratory strengthening plans and using a phased approach to implementation at the country level. Further information including prerequisites for the phased introduction of this technology can be found at: http://www.who.int/tb/publications/2008/who_htm_tb_2008_392.pdf

[6]Ibid Box 2.1.

4. WHO policy recommendations on DST of second-line anti-TB drugs
An Expert Group convened by WHO in 2007 reviewed current evidence and re-confirmed that the laboratory diagnosis of MDR-TB and XDR-TB under good laboratory practice is reliable and reproducible. In addition, this consultative process culminated in an interim policy guidance document summarizing available evidence on the second-line DST methods, and providing recommendations for which drugs to test as well as the critical concentrations. The document also provides programmatic advice on designing diagnostic algorithms, required laboratory capacity and safety requirements. The Expert Group also developed a detailed outline for the update of the 2001 technical guidelines for DST of second-line drugs, incorporating the newer technologies. A writing committee was established with the aim of releasing the updated guidelines by the middle of 2009. Policy guidance on drug-susceptibility testing (DST) of second-line anti-tuberculosis drugs can be found at: http://www.who.int/tb/publications/2008/who_

To address the challenges of implementing the changes in diagnosis of TB, WHO established the Global Laboratory Initiative (GLI) in 2007. This initiative is the part of the Stop TB Partnership, with a secretariat housed in WHO. Its major objectives include providing global standards for laboratory services, promoting quality assurance and adequate laboratory biosafety, accelerating human resource development for laboratory activities, and facilitating partnerships that will enable the establishment or expansion of laboratory services capable of absorbing new technologies. One such example is a GLI project that aims to accelerate access to new diagnostic tools for MDR-TB that have recently been endorsed by WHO. The project is being implemented in 16 of the high MDR-TB burden countries in close collaboration with the Foundation for Innovative New Diagnostics and the Global Drug Facility, with funding from UNITAID.

In the area of health system strengthening, diagnosis and treatment of TB is fully integrated into general health services in most countries. Links with general health sector or development planning frameworks are variable, but alignment with sector-wide approaches was comparatively good among reporting countries. With the expansion of the TB Technical

Assistance Mechanism known as TBTEAM (Box 6[7]), it is anticipated that technical assistance for drug management as well as many other components of TB control will be increased.

Box 6: Providing technical assistance for TB control: the role of TBTEAM

The TB Technical Assistance Mechanism, known as TBTEAM, was established by the Stop TB Partnership in 2007. TBTEAM is designed to facilitate access to high-quality, well-coordinated technical assistance, which is widely recognized as being needed to fully implement the Stop TB Strategy and the Global Plan. TBTEAM has developed a roster of experts, tools for tracking missions and training opportunities around the world, as well as a directory of technical partners. Requests for technical assistance can be sent to the TBTEAM secretariat based in WHO headquarters, either directly or via channels such as WHO country offices and TBTEAM focal points at regional and country levels.

By the end of 2008, 839 missions and events had been recorded in the TBTEAM database, and 60 of the 81 requests for technical assistance had been responded to successfully. TBTEAM has also provided financial support for 140 country missions.

A recent external assessment of TBTEAM acknowledged the service provided by TBTEAM to countries in need of technical assistance as well as its efforts to provide funding for such assistance. This assessment has also provided guidance related to the future direction of TBTEAM, including how to best engage all partners. A plan to implement the recommendations of the external assessment is being developed following broad agreement with these recommendations during a meeting of TBTEAM partners in October 2008.

Further details about TBTEAM are available at: http://www.stoptb

Pitfalls of Stop TB Strategy[8]

A much larger TB drug resistance problem exists than researchers previously thought. New global data on TB, published by WHO, highlight serious weaknesses in many national TB programmes, which increase the potential for widespread TB drug resistance. According to WHO, increasing levels of TB drug resistance reflects a failure to implement the WHO Stop TB Strategy. Some reasons identified include the following.

---

[7]Ibid Box 2.3.

[8]Bobby John and Tim France, The Sunday Tribune, New Delhi, May 6, 2007.

Today's standard test for TB relies on a technique (sputum microscopy) invented over a hundred years ago. It provides no information about drug resistance. Apparently, TB diagnosis is failing us.

National programmes rely only on single DOTS strategy which may suffer from many faults. The following points may be identified:

- Consistent lack of focus and investment;
- Chronologically weak TB diagnostic and laboratory services;
- Infrequent and incomplete TB drug resistance surveillance;
- Inadequate management of individual drug resistant TB cases; and
- Paltry TB infection control measures in health care settings.

Many TB endemic countries have failed to meet the exacting standards of the WHO strategy. DOTS was supposed to stem TB drug resistance. Because of its sloppy and unimaginative implementation, we are unable to do that.

Fighting TB "is the Responsibility of Every Citizen": Marcos Espinal[9]

Tuberculosis was thought to be under control but its visibility in the international community has changed all this. In reality, it has never been controlled properly except in some industrialized countries. The Stop TB partnership programme was launched to change the mentality that TB was a medical problem which it was not. TB is a social, political and human rights problem. It has not been controlled for decades.

Seven years ago the mentality was that TB was only the responsibility of the government. It must be stressed that fighting TB is the responsibility of every citizen. Stop TB has 500 partners, a global plan that costs $56 billion dollars (for 10 years). We hope by the end of the decade we will have new tools. But TB is a slow incidence decline disease. It is not going to go away immediately.

---

[9]The Hindu, New Delhi, November 23, 2007.

There is a gap in the global fund for the cause. The plan should be funded by endemic countries for their own backyard and by donor countries. For new tools the Bill and Melinda Gates Foundation is very committed but we need others to step up.

An Integrated Approach to HIV and TB

The incidence of TB among HIV patients is quite high in sub-Saharan Africa and is growing in South-East Asia. Undoubtedly TB is the number one cause of mortality among people living with HIV/AIDS. There is a strong need for actions that can prevent this. AIDS programmes can work with TB programmes to reduce the burden of TB among people living with HIV and vice versa. Access to antiretrovirals should be scaled up.

The HIV epidemic is growing in India. So this is the time to do the prevention, to start scaling up testing for HIV among TB patients, to be more open about the fact that the two diseases are working together secretly and slowly.

The case in Asia is more complex because of the population growth. Africa has the highest per capita rates of TB but the highest absolute numbers are in Asia. India is one of the top three high burden countries and population growth is huge. The TB programme is one of the best. But the awareness about TB in the country has to be promoted to acceptable levels where it can make some dent in the prevalence of the disease. TB can be cured by participation of the community, faith-based organisations, sport clubs, the private sector. We need to make sure we educate people and convince the community to participate. Health systems are weak, infrastructure is not available widely, there are areas in India and Africa where people have to walk a long way to get to the health services. Convincing the community leaders, the tribes, the society, and the community is the most important.

Case of Bangladesh: A Novel Approach to TB Control[10]

Plagued by years of sluggish governance, Bangladesh has come up with a novel innovation to curb the disease[10]. Private groups

---

[10]Somini Sengupta, The Indian Express, New Delhi, April 6, 2007.

have stepped in to take charge of the national tuberculosis treatment programme. The largest effort, run by the Bangladesh Rural Advancement, deploys an army of housewives across the country. They conduct daily household surveys in their neighbourhoods, hunt for patients who have been coughing for more than three weeks, coax them to get tested and, administer a long and rigorous treatment.

This has paid off. The detection rate in Bangladesh inched up to more than 70 percent in 2006 and the cure rate of 89 percent. They are a doorstep away from whoever supervised the treatment. They do not need to walk for hours or spend money for buses or rickshaws to get to treatment, and this largely contributes to the high cure rate. A survey showed that as much as 80 percent of tuberculosis patients in Bangladesh now received treatment from community-based approaches.

To help ensure that patients stay in treatment, the health workers collect a deposit. At the end of six months of treatment it is made sure that the last test is carried out. The deposit is returned when the patients is found clear of the disease.

WHO Plan[11]

Because of concerns over the rising incidence of drug resistance in TB patients, WHO has announced a new two-year, $2.15 billion plan to prevent, treat and control such cases. If fully implemented, several drug-resistant tuberculosis cases, including many in India, could be prevented and the lives of more than 1.2 million patients saved. The new plan outlines steps to increase the number of TB laboratories in countries with high levels of TB so that detection and treatment of resistant cases can be increased ten-fold.

The Global MDR-TB and XDR-TB Response Plan 2007-2008 of the WHO, details the steps required to provide access to drugs and diagnostic tests for all drug-resistant TB patients by 2015, and identifies costs, milestones and priorities for health services.

WHO's effort to raise awareness about TB was augmented recently at a political meet. A global campaign designated 'Call

---

[11]Amrita Nair-Ghaswalla, Times of India, New Delhi, August 16, 2007.

to Stop TB' was signed jointly by a delegation of British members of Parliament and the Indian Medical Parliamentary Forum[12]. Determined to raise the profile of tuberculosis in Westminster, the British MPs were keen to work with their colleagues in other countries to persuade governments to step up the fight against TB. They were of the view that while there was a lot of interest in the UK about AIDS, there was not equal interest about TB.

The re-emergence of tuberculosis in Britain was considered to be a consequence of immigration. People from high-burden countries have been passing on the infection. The possible link between immigration and TB was a matter of concern for decision makers particularly because the disease was completely curable.

Time to Finance a New Global Health Fund[13]

World leaders meeting at the United Nations in September 2010 were to consider accelerating progress towards the millennium development goals (MDGs). Three of the eight MDGs aim at providing primary health services to the entire world's population. The key step was to expand the Global Fund to Fight AIDS, tuberculosis and malaria into a Global Health Fund.

The Global Fund was created in 2002 to fight AIDS, tuberculosis and malaria. Its implementation and management made it the most successful innovation in foreign assistance of the past decade. The achievements include putting an estimated 2.5 million people on anti-retroviral AIDS therapy, curing about eight million people of tuberculosis and distributing more than 100 million long-lasting insecticide-treated bed nets to fight against malaria. These efforts resulted in saving of an estimated five million lives.

Since 2002, the Global Fund has approved around $19 billion in funding. However, the Fund is facing two huge challenges. The first is lack of financing. Because of its success, countries are submitting increasingly ambitious programmes for

[12]British MPs keen to raise TB profile in Westminster, The Tribune, New Delhi,29 March 2007.

[13]The Economic Times, New Delhi, 22 March 2010.

consideration. Unfortunately, the Global Fund is already in a state of fiscal crisis. It needs around $6 billion per year in the next three years to cover expansion of programmes for the three diseases, but it has only around $3 billion per year from donor countries.

The second challenge is to broaden the Global Fund's mandate. So far, the Global Fund has addressed MDG 6, which is focused on the control of specific killer diseases. The control of these three diseases inevitably involves improvement of basic health services which play a fundamental role in achieving MDG 4 (reduction of child mortality) and MDG 5 (reduction of maternal mortality). All three health MDGs are interconnected; all are feasible with an appropriate scaling up of primary health services. This will, however, require expansion of the Global Fund's financing mandate to include financing for training and deployment of community health workers, construction and operation of local health facilities, and other components of primary health systems.

Many countries have recently recognized the need to move beyond the financing of control of AIDS, tuberculosis and malaria to financing improvements in primary health systems more generally. But they seem to view the issue of health-system financing as an either-or choice: scale up control of AIDS, tuberculosis and malaria, or scale up financing of primary health systems.

The annual cost of specific disease control in the next three years is perhaps $6 billion, and another $6 billion per year for health-system expansion. The total, $12 billion per year for an expanded Global Fund, might seem unrealistically-large compared to the $3 billion per year spent now. But total annual funding of $12 billion is really very modest, representing around 0.033% (three cents per $100) of the donor countries' GNP.

If the US would expand its annual support to the Global Fund to around $4 billion per year, it would likely induce the rest of the world's donors to put in $8 billion per year, keeping the US share at around a third of the total funding.

4.3 CASE OF INDIA

Tuberculosis control has always been the concern of the Government of India and several NGOs for almost half a century. A National Tuberculosis Programme (NTP), aimed at controlling the disease, was established in India in 1962, a long time before the launch of currently revised programme. The infrastructure and awareness raising achieved during almost three decades of NTP helped the smooth launch of RNTCP, wherein for the first time a concerted effort was being made to reach the patients at all India level. Further, the selection of the DOTS centre was according to the patients convenience (closer to their residence) so that they did not lose wages or incur transportation charges for treatment under the programme. RNTCP uses the most systematic and cost-effective approach, has the political and the administrative commitment to (i) ensure the provision of organized and comprehensive TB Control Services; (ii) reliable and early diagnosis through smear microscopy of self reporting chest symptomatics in the general health services; (iii) an uninterrupted supply of good quality anti-TB drugs; (iv) an effective and patient -friendly treatment; and (v) systematic monitoring as well as accountability[14].

In view of the huge economic, social and health etc., costs and increasing burden of tuberculosis, India launched the Revised National Tuberculosis Control Programme (RNTCP) on a pilot basis in 1993, using the universally adopted Directly Observed Treatment Short Course (DOTS) recommended by WHO. This strategy, currently being used by 200 of the 211 countries world wide reporting to WHO, is one of the largest public health programmes found to be beneficial in the world. This strategy has been successful in reducing death rates and increasing cure rates throughout, including India. The success is largely ascribed to the sound technical elements of the strategy including (i) case detection through quality-assured

[14]SP Agarwal, Sophia Vijay, P Kumar, LS Chauhan, The History of Tuberculosis Control in India: Glimpses through Decades, in Tuberculosis Control in India, SP Agarwal and LS Chauhan (eds.),Directorate General of Health Services, Ministry of Health and Family Welfare, New Delhi, 2006.

bacteriology, (ii) standardized treatment with supervision and patient support, (iii) an effective drug supply and management system, and (iv) monitoring and evaluation system and impact measurement[15].

Large-scale implementation of RNTCP, however, began only in 1997. The initial five-year project, with assistance from the World Bank, was to implement the programme in 102 districts of the country, and strengthen facilities in additional 203 districts for introduction of the revised strategy at a later stage. In early 2002, the World Bank- assisted TB control project was extended for another two years, within the same budgetary provision, to cover a population of 700 million. The Government of India, however, took up the challenge of nationwide expansion of RNTCP by the year 2005, and before the start of the next phase of the project[16].

RNTCP in India is the second largest programme in the world and is integrated with primary health care services. India has an extensive network of primary health centers (PHCs) and they are involved in all the public health programmes including tuberculosis[17].

The second phase of RNTCP was launched in October 2006 where; besides continuing the ongoing work further, widening services and sustaining them over a long period of time; emphasis was placed on the treatment of multidrug resistant TB through DOTS-Plus treatment. During the current phase, wider collaboration with other sectors aims to provide standardized, good quality treatment and diagnostic services to all patients in a patient-friendly environment, irrespective of the health care facility from which they seek treatment.

[15]WHO: Global Tuberculosis Control: Surveillance, Planning, Financing. WHO Report 2006, Geneva, World Health Organization (WHO/HTM/TB/2006.362), p. 18.

[16]TB India 2006, RNTCP Status Report, Central TB Division,). Directorate General of Health Services, Ministry of Health and Family Welfare, New Delhi, p.16.

[17]M Muniyandi, Rajeswari R, R Balasubramanian, Estimating provider cost for treating patient with tuberculosis under Revised National Tuberculosis Control Programme (RNTCP) Tuberculosis Research Centre (ICMR), Chennai. p. 2.

The basic principles of the RNTCP are:

- Political and administrative commitment to ensure adequate funds, staff and other key inputs for organized and comprehensive TB control services.
- Reliable and early diagnosis through smear microscopy of self reporting chest symptomatics in the general health services.
- Regular and uninterrupted supply of anti-TB medications including the use of a patient-wise box which contains the entire course of treatment for an individual patient so that no patient should ever stop treatment for lack of medicines;
- Effective and patient-friendly environment and direct observation of every dose of treatment in the intensive phase and at least the first dose in the continuation phase of treatment; and
- Systematic monitoring, supervision and cohort analysis. One senior treatment Supervisor for organization of uninterrupted treatment and one senior tuberculosis Laboratory Supervisor for ensuring quality laboratory service for every 5 lakh population. Additional staff is provided for difficult hilly, tribal, and some urban areas.

If three AFB smears are negative and there is no response to 1–2 weeks of antibiotics, X-ray is taken and, if consistent with TB, the patient is treated for smear-negative TB. If only one of three specimens is positive, an X-ray is taken and the patient is evaluated. All treatments are given thrice weekly on alternate days. During the intensive phase, every dose is directly observed; medications for the continuation phase are packaged into a weekly blister pack, at least the first dose of which is directly observed.

Policy direction, supervision, drugs and microscopes are provided by the Central Government. Districts receive funds directly from the Central Government out of the World Bank, Danida, or DFID assistance. The funds are released to hire contractual staff, conduct training, POL, IEC, purchase of vehicles and other items essential for performing functions efficiently. Printed technical and operational guidelines have been provided to all health centers, laboratory guidelines have been provided to all microscopy centre, and illustrated guidelines for health providers giving observed treatment have been provided in local languages. Modular training has been used for all staff from medical officers to health workers. Multi-purpose workers are responsible for treatment observation; where they are not available, treatment observation is done by community volunteers including Anganwadi workers, traditional dais, and community and religious leaders. Observation by a family member is not acceptable in the programme. In some larger cities with limited health infrastructure, the RNTCP has funded specialized, full-time staff for microscopy and for treatment observation.

Perhaps the greatest strength of the RNTCP is the new recording and reporting system. This system ensures accountability for each and every patient begun on treatment. The programme is entirely open to a frank and fair analysis of the data, and to objective evaluation of alternative strategies which might improve the quality of diagnosis and/or treatment and/or compliance. Case detection rates have been high, quality of diagnosis has been relatively good, and sputum conversion rates remain high.

Targets for RNTCP

The goal of RNTCP is to cure at least 85% of new smear-positive cases of tuberculosis and to detect at least 70% of such patients, after the desired cure rate has been achieved. Both the goals are desirable, but it is imperative that the system is geared-up to reliably cure patients first and then to expand case detection. The advantage of this approach is logically based on the experience that reliably curing patients leads to a "recruitment effect" — wherever effective services are offered, case detection rates steadily increase. Cured patients act as one of the best motivators and promote case detection and patient adherence to treatment.

RNTCP in India has adopted the targets set by WHO (Box 1) and the strategy. Expansion and enhancement of high quality DOTS services is considered the key component of a comprehensive strategy to achieve the targets set above. The programme uses the following system:

- An individual box of medications for the entire duration of treatment is earmarked for every patient registered. This ensures the availability of the medicines for the full course of treatment to each registered patient.
- A health worker or another trained person who is not a family member, watches as the patient swallows the anti-TB medicines in her/his presence. RNTCP uses Short Course Chemotherapy (SCC) regimes, which reduces the duration of treatment and facilitates directly observed treatment.
- Health provider ensures that the right drugs in the right doses are taken at right intervals for the right duration.

Treatment under DOTS leads to 85–95% success rate whereas that without observation can give only as estimated 50–60% success rate.

Advantages of DOTS

1. Accuracy of TB diagnosis is more than doubled.
2. Treatment success rate is up to 95%.
3. Prevents spread of the tuberculosis bacillus, thus reducing the incidence and prevalence of TB.
4. Helps alleviate poverty by saving lives, reducing duration of illness and preventing spread of infection.
5. Improves quality of health care and removes stigma associated with TB.
6. Prevents failure of treatment and the emergence of multidrug resistant-TB by ensuring patient adherence and uninterrupted drug supply.
7. Lends credibility to TB control effects.
8. Provides a model for strengthening health services.
9. Selects DOTS centre in according to patient's convenience (closer to patient's residence) so that patients do not lose wages or incur transportation charges for treatment in the programme.
10. Uses all possible treatment outcomes such as cure, treatment completed, defaulted, failure, transferred out and death defined as given below.

Cured is a case who was initially smear-positive, who has completed treatment and has negative sputum smears, on at least two occasions, one of which was at the completion of treatment.

Treatment completed is a sputum smear-positive case who has completed treatment, with negative smear at the end of the initial phase but none at the end of treatment, or a sputum smear-negative TB patient who has received a full course of treatment and has not become smear-positive during or at the end of treatment, or an extra-pulmonary TB patient who had received a full course of treatment and has not become smear-positive during or at the end of treatment.

Default is a patient who, at any time after registration, has not taken anti-TB drugs for 2 or more consecutive months.

Transferred out is a patient who has been transferred to another tuberculosis unit/district and whose treatment results are not known.

Death a patient who died during the treatment, regardless of cause

Failure is a smear-positive case which is smear-positive at 5 months or more after starting treatment. Also refers to a patient who was initially smear-negative and treated in category III, but who became smear-positive during treatment.

Progress of DOTS in India

We have used two data sources to assess the progress of TB control in India. The data from WHO help us to assess the progress of TB control in India and compare that with progress achieved in selected groups of countries of our interest. In the context of TB, and for comparative purposes, the selected groups identified are those that form the High Burden Countries (HBCs), South East Asia Region (SEAR) consisting of the countries in this region and the Global level that comprises all the countries for which WHO collects data. On the other hand, data from official sources help us to assess the progress as reported by the Central TB Division (CTD), Government of India, and compare the same with that given by WHO for India. These groups of countries are not mutually exclusive and India is a constituent in each of these.

International Perspective

The progress of the implementation of RNTCP in India has been quite rapid. Starting on a pilot basis in October 1993 and covering a population of 2.35 million, it expanded to cover about 18 million people by 1998. Thereafter, the Programme expanded dramatically and by the years 2000, 2002 and 2004 it covered 30%, 50% and 87% of the country's population. By the end of December 2005, it covered a population of 1,080 million or 97% of the total population of the country in the year and was spread in 616 districts of 35 states/union Territories. By March 2006, the entire country was covered by the DOTS system.

In view of the targets set by WHO under its Stop TB Strategy it would be useful to examine the progress made by DOTS approach. Three parameters have been identified to gauge this progress. These are (1) percentage of population covered by DOTS (coverage rate), (2) percentage of new smear-positive TB cases detected (the detection rate) and (3) the percentage of those cured/completed treatment among the ones registered for treatment and detected as new smear-positive cases (the success rate). Success is defined to include those cases classified as cured as well as those who completed the treatment but cure could not be confirmed by laboratory tests. The trend in the progress made by DOTS strategy as measured with the help of these three parameters over the years since the launch of the programme in India is presented below. The trend in India is compared with that in High Burden Countries (HBCs), South East Asia Region (SEAR) and the Global total.

Coverage of Population by DOTS Strategy

According to the WHO Report for 2008, the total number of countries implementing DOTS increased rapidly since 1995 and approached 184 of 211 in 2006. By the year 2000 each of the 22 HBCs had established the DOTS programme. As such by the end of 2006, 93% of the world's population was living in political/administrative areas that had adopted DOTS strategy. In 2006 the coverage by DOTS was reported more than 90% for five of the six regions in which the WHO classified the countries. It varied between 91% for Africa to 100% for South

East Asia Region and West Pacific Region. The coverage rate for Europe was surprisingly very low at 67% in 2006[18].

At the global level the coverage DOTS programme increased steadily since 1995. It increased from 22% in 1995 to 93% in 2006. Similar trend for progress in coverage rate may be noted in the case of India, HBCs and SEAR. Though slightly better than the global rate in 2004, the coverage of population by DOTS programme in India at 84% was poorer than that for all the HBCs (87%) and for SEAR (89%) (Table 4.1). The situation, however, changed radically thereafter and by 2006 with 100% coverage India succeeded in providing DOTS facility to its entire population, the same as the South East Asia Region.

Table 4.1: Progress in coverage rate for DOTS implementation by specified country/region and year, 1995–2006

SPECIFIED AREAS

Year	*India*	*High-burden Countries*	*South East Asian region*	*Global*
Percentage of total population covered by DOTS*				
1995	1.5	24	6.6	22
1996	2	32	12	32
1997	2.3	36	16	37
1998	9	43	29	43
1999	13.5	45	36	47
2000	30	55	49	57
2001	45	61	60	62
2002	51.6	68	66	69
2003	67.2	79	77	78
2004	84.0	87	89	83
2005	91.0	94	93	89
2006	100	98	100	93

Source: WHO Report 2008 Global Tuberculosis Control, Surveillance, Planning Financing, Table: 2.5, p. 41.

*Percentage of the national population living in areas where health services have opted DOTS. (Areas here are the lowest administrative or management units in the country).

[18]WHO: Global Tuberculosis Control: Surveillance, Planning, Financing. WHO Report 2008, Geneva, World Health. Organization, Table 2.5, p.41.

Compared to HBCs, the DOTS programme in India made an accelerated progress where coverage rate increased from a very low level of 1.5% in 1995 to 84% in 2004. The acceleration may be noted to start after the year 2000.

Case Detection Rate

The case detection rate of new smear-positive TB cases (%) from DOTS programme, because of recent implementation, was very low and varied marginally between 0.3% and 1.6% during 1995 and 1998. By contrast, the detection rate for the country as a whole was quite high and comparable to global rates in those years varying between 37% and 40%. The detection rate began accelerating after 1998, with acceleration much faster for DOTS areas than that for the whole country and the gap eventually disappearing by the year 2006. This implies that the progress in overall detection rate in the country was largely the result of the improvements in RNTCP through DOTS (Table 4.2). Somewhat similar trend in the detection rate with negligible differential between DOTS and the total areas may be noted at the global level as well as for, HBCs and SEAR. It is significant to note that the detection rate at the country level for India has consistently remained slightly higher than that at the global level as well as that for the HBCs. The SEAR shows the reverse of this pattern after 2004 (Table 4.2).

The preceding observation, however, is not valid for DOTS programme. Because of its recent origin, the level of detection rate under the DOTS in India remained consistently lower than that in other areas including the global level all along until 2002. Thereafter, with accelerated expansion, the level of detection rate in India caught up to global as well as other area levels. India experienced a marginally higher detection rate than HBCs and global level but it still fell short of the rate for SEAR. The detection rate under DOTS programme in India started at 0.3% in 1995, increased gradually until 2000 before accelerating to 64% by 2006. It may be noted that the case detection rate under DOTS showed a slow progress even globally, though at a higher level than that in India, from 11% in 1995 to 37% in 2002. It accelerated thereafter and reached a level of 61% in 2006.

Table 4.2: Case detection rate of new smear-positive cases (%) by specified area, type of programme and year, 1995–2006

SPECIFIED AREAS

Year	*India*		*High-Burden Countries*		*South East Asia Region*		*Global Total*	
	DOTS Programme	*Whole Country*	*DOTS Programme*	*Whole Country*	*DOTS Programme*	*Whole Country*	*DOTS Programme*	*Whole Country*
1995	0.3	37	8.3	31	1.5	29	11	35
1996	0.9	40	14	36	4.0	30	16	39
1997	1.0	37	16	37	5.5	29	18	40
1998	1.6	37	20	37	8.0	30	22	41
1999	6.8	45	23	39	14	37	24	42
2000	12	44	26	39	18	39	28	41
2001	23	48	30	40	27	42	32	43
2002	30	49	34	42	34	45	37	44
2003	43	52	43	47	44	50	44	49
2004	55	58	53	55	55	57	52	55
2005	59	60	59	60	62	62	58	60
2006	64	64	63	63	67	67	61	62

Source: WHO, op.cit.,Table 1.4, p. 25.

Note: DOTS case detection rate = $\frac{\text{Annual new smear-positive notifications (DOTS)}}{\text{Estimated annual smear positive incidence (country)}}$

For finding the case detection rate for the country, the numerator in the above formula is replaced by the comparable number for the country.

Treatment Success Rate

Globally 1.712 million new-smear-positive cases were registered for treatment in DOTS programme in 2003[19]. The number increased to 2.359 million two years later for the cohort of 2005. The cure rate among all cases under DOTS for cohort registered in 2003 was 75%. An additional 7% completed the treatment but were not confirmed for cure by laboratory tests. Thus, the reported treatment success rate was 82%[20]. The cure rate went up to 78% for the cohort of 2005 and consequently the success rate became 85%[21].The treatment success rate globally for DOTS programme remained between 77% for 1994 and 1996 cohort and 82% for cohort of 2000 through 2003 increasing thereafter slowly to reach a level of 85% for the cohort of 2005 (Table 4.3). For the first time in the history of DOTS the global success rate reached the target set by WHO for the cohort registered for treatment in 2005.

As far as success rate is concerned, the achievement of DOTS programme in India has been somewhat better than that at global level for each annual cohort registered for treatment during the period considered here. The rate for India ranged between 79% for cohort of 1995, 1996 and 87% for the cohort of 2002. India has achieved and even bettered the target rate of 85% for five consecutive cohorts of 2001 through 2005, the slight dip of one percentage point in success rate for cohort of 2003 through 2005 as compared to that for cohort of 2002 could be due to rapid expansion in the programme. The success rate for India has been somewhat better than that for HBCs consistently for each cohort registered during 1996 to 2003. Similar observation may be noted for achievement of DOTS programme in India vis–a–vis that in SEAR. However, the success rate for India for cohorts of 2004 and 2005 were equal to that for HBCs and a percentage point lower than that for SEAR. It may be noted that the success rate in India appears to have stabilized at the target level set for the programme. In future this has to be kept-up and improved. Details are given in Table 4.3.

[19]WHO Report for 2006, Table 9, p. 39.
[20]Ibid., Table 10, p. 40.
[21]WHO Report for 2008, Table 1.5, p. 29.

Table 4.3: Treatment success rate for new-smear-positive cases (%) by specified areas, type of programme and year of contact of patients, 1994–2005

SPECIFIED AREAS

Year of Cohort	*India*		*High-Burden*		*South East Asia Region*		*Global*	
	DOTS Programme	*Whole Country*	*DOTS Programme*	*Whole Country*	*DOTS Programme*	*Whole Country*	*DOTS Programme*	*Whole Country*
1994	83	*	87	83	80	66	77	75
1995	79	25	83	53	74	33	79	57
1996	79	21	78	50	77	31	77	54
1997	82	18	81	56	72	29	79	60
1998	84	27	83	62	72	40	81	64
1999	82	21	81	60	73	34	80	64
2000	84	34	84	67	83	50	82	69
2001	85	54	84	72	84	63	82	73
2002	87	60	83	75	85	68	82	76
2003	86	76	84	80	85	79	83	80
2004	86	–	86	–	87	–	84	–
2005	86	–	86	–	87	–	85	–

Source: WHO, Report for 2008, Table 1.6, p. 30.

The high levels of treatment success rate achieved under DOTS strategy globally as well as in India are commendable, particularly because the number of patients covered by the programme has been rising rapidly. Globally the number increased from 240,000 in 1994 to 1.7 million in 2003 and further to 2.5 million in 2005. For India, the number of patients notified/registered for treatment under DOTS increased from 185,000 in 2001 to 359,000 in 2003 and further to 506,000 in 2005.

Comparison of Estimates for DOTS Progress Given by WHO and RNTCP Status Reports

Study based on data given by WHO shows substantial progress in tuberculosis control through implementation of DOTS strategy. Similar conclusion may be reached by analyzing the data released by CTD, DGHS, MOHFW, GoI. However, when we compare the two data sets, substantial quantitative and sometimes confusing differences are noted. This comparison is attempted in Table 4.4.

Table 4.4: Comparison of progress of DOTS programme in India as given by WHO and the RNTCP status reports for specified years

Year of registration	*Coverage Rate (%)*		*Detection Rate (%)*		*Year of Cohort*	*Success Rate (%)*	
	*WHO**	*RNTCP*	*WHO**	*RNTCP*		*WHO**	*RNTCP*
2001	45	44**	24	56	2000	84	84
2002	51.6	51**	31	59	2001	85	85
2003	67.2	73**	45	69	2002	87	87
2004	84	87***	57	72	2003	86	86
2005	91	97***	59	66	2004	86	86
2006	100	100	64	66	2005	86	86

Notes: *WHO figures are given in Tables 4.1, 4.2 and 4.3 given above.
**Calculated by using the population covered given in RNTCP Status Report and the estimated population of India for respective years.
***Figures are taken from the Annual Report of RNTCP.
Source: Respective RNTCP Status Reports.

Both data sets show substantial progress in coverage of population for TB control under DOTS. However, WHO estimates for the year 2003, 2004 and 2005 at 67%, 84% and

91% respectively are lower than CTD estimates at 73%, 87% and 97%. This difference of 6, 3 and 6 percentage points is hard to reconcile. Both sources, however, agree at the estimated coverage rate at 100% by 2006.

The differences between the coverage rates by the two data sources turn out to be minor when compared to those in detection rate. The estimates of the detection rate given by WHO are substantially lower than those given by CTD except for the year 2006. The differences decline with passage of time. For example, for the year 2001, WHO estimate at 24% was less than one-half of that given by CTD (56%), a gap of 32 percentage points. The difference declines to 15 percentage points in 2004 after keeping high values of 28 and 24 points in 2002 and 2003. The difference declined precipitously and stood at 7 and 2 percentage points for 2005 and 2006 respectively. The basic reason for this difference lies in the definition of the denominator of the rate. The report from CTD apparently uses the population of the areas covered by the programme to arrive at the estimated total number of new smear-positive cases for the programme areas and computes the detection rate. By contrast, WHO uses the estimated number of new smear-positive cases for the whole country in the denominator. In brief the detection rate given by WHO is for the whole country and is therefore comparable to similar rate for any other country-level data whereas the rate given by RNTCP is for the areas served by the DOTS programme and is not comparable to figures that represent the country. The rates calculated by the RNTCP may be used for the evaluation of the programme but serve limited purpose for international comparability of the performance. It may be pointed out here that with 100% coverage by DOTS, the coverage rates given by WHO and RNTCP are expected to be identical. The possibility is demonstrated by the declining trend in the difference of detection rates given by the two sources.

National Perspectives: Performance of RNTCP in Different States/Union Territories of India

India presents a complex picture of heterogeneity with regard to several characteristics. These differences get reflected, among other things, in the performance achieved by various development and other projects. It may be interesting to examine whether such differences are likely to extend to the performance of RNTCP as well. The states and union Territories being important administrative divisions of the country are considered to study these variations in implementation of DOTS Programme.

The two important parameters to measure the performance of DOTS are detection rate for new smear-positive TB cases and success rate for cure/completion of treatment among those registered. The analysis of the performance by administrative divisions, namely, states and union territories, may be useful in highlighting the areas where more action would be needed to improve the functioning of the programme. The data used here are taken from the RNTCP Status Reports issued by the Central TB Division, Directorate General of Health Services (DGHS), Ministry of Health and Family Welfare (MOHFEW), Government of India (GOI) for the years 2001 through 2007. Since the Programme has been through expansion phase over the years, these data relating to different years are available only for those states where the Programme was in operation in that year. We noted earlier that RNTCP covered 100% of the population for the first time by March 2006. Also, the same year, the data on the performance in respect of the detection and success rates were made available, for the first time, for 35 states/union Territories. The achievements of different states/union Territories showed wide variability. It may be noted that in 2007 the success rate, with reference to national average rate of 86%, varied within a narrow range of 71% for Lakshdweep and 92% for Daman and Diu. By contrast, the detection rate with reference to national average of 66% varied widely between 12% for Lakshdweep and 112% for Sikkim.

The distribution of the states/union territories over the years 2001 to 2005 by performance in respect of detection and success rates with reference to whether these met or missed the target set by WHO is summarized in Table 4.5. The table presents the classification of states/union territories where the data for both the detection and success rates are given in four different categories according to performance. These categories are:

- **UADS:** states/union Territories which failed to achieve the target for detection rate as well as for success rate.
- **UAD:** states/union Territories which failed to achieve the detection rate but were able to achieve the required success rate.
- **UAS:** states/union Territories which failed to achieve the required success rate but were able to achieve the detection rate.
- **ADS:** states/union Territories which achieved the target for both the detection rate and the success rate.

Combination of categories UADS and UAD helps us to identify all those states/union Territories which under achieved on detection rate whereas the similar operation on categories UADS and UAS lists the areas considered here which under achieved on the success rate.

Table 4.5: Distribution of states/union territories implementing DOTS programme by performance status 2001–05, India

Year	*Performance status*				
	UADS	*UAD*	*UAS*	*ADS*	*N*
2001	9	5	2	2	18
2002	7	5	2	5	19
2003	3	12	2	8	25
2004	6	8	2	11	27
2005	7	13	1	10	31
2006	11	11	3	10	35
2007	7	12	1	15	35

Source: Compiled from Table 4.8.

It may be obtained from Table 4.5 that states/union territories which failed to achieve the target in respect of detection rate in different years from 2001 to 2007, respectively, numbered 14 of 18 (78%), 12 of 19 (63%), 15 of 25 (60%), 14 of 27 (52%), 20 of 31 (65%), 22 of 35 (63%) and 19 of 35 (54%). Thus, more than one-half of the states/union Territories where the prgramme was operational fell short of target as far as detection rate was concerned. The high occurrence of under performance particularly in respect of detection rate, a key indicator in the success of RNTCP, needs to be addressed to improve the overall performance of the Programme in the country.

To facilitate the identification of under-achievers Table 4.6 lists the states/union Territories in ascending order of detection rate within each performance category for the entire period considered here. Similar classification with reference to success rate had not been attempted because of limited variability in this rate from one administrative area identified here to another.

Here, it is useful to examine the extent of variability in detection and success rates over various years in different states and union territories. Table 4.7 summarizes the findings and reveals considerable variation in the two rates. At the national level the achievement appears quite satisfactory where the target for both the indicators was achieved in 2007. This, as expected, hides wide variability in both the indicators when examined at state and union territory levels. We may note that, in general, the range of variation for success rate was narrower than that for detection rate. Further, it was narrower for major states than that for all states/union territories taken together. Major states showed some sort of stability in the range lying between 10 and 13 points. By contrast, the range of variation in success rate for extended unites considered here was between 11 and 30. As opposed to this, the detection rate among major states varied between 37 and 63 and among all areas between 46 and 102. Whereas the range of variation for success rate showed stability over the years that for detection rate, particularly for all areas, showed a rising trend reaching as high as 102 in 2006.

Further, to improve the performance of DOTS in different states/union territories, it is useful to identify the states which either under perform or slip to this category more often than others. To this end the annual performance data summarized in Table 4.8 were re-examined with reference to states for which the detection and success rates were reported for each year over the period of 2001–2007. There were 18 states in this category. The performance of these states is summarized in

Table 4.6: Classification of states and union territories according to level of achieving the target in respect of detection rate for new smear-positive TB cases and success rate among the registered case: India, 2001-07, Areas in each category group are arranged in ascending order of detection rate

2001		*2002*		*2003*		*2004*		*2005*		*2006*		*2007*	
Under achievers for both the detection and success rates													
Tamil Nadu	45	Punjab	38	Chhattisgarh	47	Uttar Pradesh	54	Meghalaya	50	Bihar	27	Lakshadweep	12
Jharkhand	47	West Bengal	51	Haryana	57	Nagaland	55	Goa	53	Jammu & Kashmir	33	Bihar	45
Maharashtra	48	Madhya Pradesh	54	Gujarat	66	Madhya Pradesh	60	Madhya Pradesh	53	Kerala	43	Goa	51
Gujarat	53	Gujarat	57			Karnataka	65	Assam	55	Goa	52	Karnataka	61
West Bengal	53	Tamil Nadu	59			Orissa	65	Haryana	57	Madhya Pradesh	54	D&N Haveli	62
Madhya Pradesh	55	Karnataka	62			Meghalaya	67	Orissa	60	Punjab	55	Kerala	64
Haryana	56	Haryana	64					Karnataka	63	Karnataka	60	Tamil Nadu	68
Andhra Pradesh	56									Haryana	60		
Karnataka	61									Assam	64		
										Meghalaya	66		
										Tamil Nadu	68		

Contd...

Table 4.6: Classification of states and union territories according to level of achieving the target in respect of detection rate for new smear-positive TB cases and success rate among the registered case: India, 2001-07, Areas in each category group are arranged in ascending order of detection rate (*Contd...*)

2001		*2002*		*2003*		*2004*		*2005*		*2006*		*2007*	
Under achievers for detection rate but not for success rate													
Bihar	37	Bihar	47	Punjab	41	Kerala	45	Jammu & Kashmir	25	Lakshad-weep	14	Jammu & Kashmir	43
Kerala	60	Maharashtra	50	Uttaranchal	44	Bihar	49	Bihar	27	Tripura	49	Manipur	55
Himachal Pradesh	61	Jharkhand	59	Kerala	45	Punjab	50	Tripura	40	Uttaranchal	49	Madhya Pradesh	56
Uttar Pradesh	67	Kerala	63	Nagaland	47	Uttaranchal	61	Kerala	45	Uttar Pradesh	52	Punjab	56
Rajasthan	69	Himachal Pradesh	65	Bihar	48	Chhattisgarh	62	Punjab	48	Manipur	59	Uttar Pradesh	56
				Uttar Pradesh	55	Jharkhand	63	Uttar Pradesh	49	Orissa	59	Tripura	56
				Jharkhand	55	Maharashtra	67	Jharkhand	50	Chhattisgarh	59	Chhattisgarh	57
				Madhya Pradesh	55	Manipur	68	Uttaranchal	51	Nagaland	60	Haryana	59
				Maharashtra	59			Manipur	53	Jharkhand	64	Uttaranchal	61
				Assam	62			Nagaland	53	Maharashtra	65	Orissa	65
				West Bengal	64			Chhattisgarh	55	Daman & Diu	67	Maharashtra	66
				Karnataka	66			Maharashtra	66			Daman & Diu	67
								Gujarat	69				

Contd...

Table 4.6: Classification of states and union territories according to level of achieving the target in respect of detection rate for new smear-positive TB cases and success rate among the registered case: India, 2001-07, Areas in each category group are arranged in ascending order of detection rate (*Contd...*)

2001		*2002*		*2003*		*2004*		*2005*		*2006*		*2007*	
Under achievers for success rate but not for detection rate													
Assam	73	Andhra Pradesh	71	Chandigarh	77	Assam	70	Pondicherry	78	D & N Haveli	75	Meghalaya	77
Delhi	79	Delhi	92	Delhi	80	Haryana	70			Pondicherry	85		
				Arunachal Pradesh	91					Andaman & Nicobar	93		
Target achievers for both the detection rate and success rate													
Manipur	82	Manipur	72	Tamil Nadu	73	West Bengal	70	Mizoram	74	Andhra Pradesh	74	Assam	74
Orissa	83	Uttar Pradesh	73	Manipur	77	Gujarat	72	Andhra	74	Gujarat	77	Chandigarh	75
		Rajasthan	76	Rajasthan	79	Chandigarh	76	West Bengal	76	Mizoram	77	Andaman & Nicobar	85
		Assam	78	Andhra Pradesh	81	Andhra Pradesh	77	Chandigarh	76	West Bengal	78	Delhi	87
		Orissa	79	Sikkim	82	Delhi	81	Rajasthan	77	Rajasthan	80	Sikkim	112
				Himachal Pradesh	82	Arunachal Pradesh	81	Tamil Nadu	77	Himachal Pradesh	81	West Bengal	77
				Orissa	91	Rajasthan	81	Himachal Pradesh	78	Chandigarh	82	Gujarat	78

Contd...

Table 4.6: Classification of states and union territories according to level of achieving the target in respect of detection rate for new smear-positive TB cases and success rate among the registered case: India, 2001-07, Areas in each category group are arranged in ascending order of detection rate (*Contd...*)

2001		*2002*		*2003*		*2004*		*2005*		*2006*		*2007*	
						Mizoram	82	Delhi	83	Delhi	90	Andhra Pradesh	81
						Himachal Pradesh	82	Arunachal Pradesh	89	Arunachal Pradesh	105	Arunachal Pradesh	100
						Tamil Nadu	82	Sikkim	115	Sikkim	116	Jharkhand	73
						Sikkim	125					Himachal Pradesh	81
												Rajasthan	81
												Nagaland	74
												Pondicherry	80
												Mizoram	95
N	**18**		**19**		**25**		**27**		**31**		**35**		**35**

Table 4.7: Range of variation for success rate (SR) and detection rate (DR) with corresponding names, along with lowest and highest values for all states and union territories and major states in India

2001		2002		2003		2004		2005		2006		2007	
RANGE ANALYSIS FOR SR													
SR India	**84**		**85**		**87**		**86**		**86**		**86**		**86**
All states and union territories													
Gujarat	78	Andhra	81	Chandigarh	80	Meghalaya	76	Pondicherry	75	Goa	70	Lakshadweep	71
Himachal	90	Bihar	92	Uttaranchal	95	Jharkhand	93	Arunachal	97	Lakshadweep	100	Daman & Diu	92
Range	**12**		**11**		**15**		**17**		**22**		**30**		**21**
Major states only													
Gujarat	78	Andhra	81	Chhattisgarh	82	Karnataka	81	Assam	80	Karnataka	79	Karnataka	78
Himachal	90	Bihar	92	Uttaranchal	95	Jharkhand	93	Jharkhand	90	Himachal	89	Uttaranchal	89
Range	**12**		**11**		**13**		**12**		**10**		**10**		**11**
RANGE ANALYSIS FOR DR													
DR India	**56**		**59**		**69**		**72**		**66**		**66**		**70**
All states and union territories													
Bihar	37	Punjab	38	Punjab	41	Kerala	45	J & K	25	Lakshadweep	14	Lakshadweep	12
Orissa	83	Delhi	92	Orissa	91	Sikkim	125	Sikkim	115	Sikkim	116	Sikkim	112
Range	**46**		**54**		**50**		**80**		**90**		**102**		**100**
Major states only													
Bihar	37	Punjab	38	Punjab	41	Kerala	45	J & K	25	Bihar	27	J & K	43
Orissa	83	Delhi	92	Orissa	91	Himachal	82	Delhi	83	Delhi	90	Delhi	87
Range	**46**		**54**		**50**		**37**		**58**		**63**		**44**

top panel of Table 4.8. It may be noted that 3 of the 18 states listed in the top panel of Table 4.8 consistently under-performed on both the counts every year during 2001–07 except negligible instances when the target was barely met. These are: Haryana, Karnataka and Madhya Pradesh. Haryana just made the target for detection rate in 2004 but failed to meet the target for success rate in that year. In addition, this state just met the target for success rate in 2007 but failed to meet the target for detection rate. By comparison Karnataka and Madhya Pradesh failed to meet the target for detection rate year after year during the period 2001–07 but could barely manage to meet the target for success rate in 2003 (both) and in 2007 (only Karnataka). Thus, it may be noted that the detection rate in these three states was perpetually below the target. The departure for detection rate from the target in Madhya Pradesh was more than that in Karnataka and Haryana and generally reached as high as 14 to 17 percentage points. By comparison, this departure for Karnataka was between 1 to 10 percentage points. In addition, other states which substantially under-performed on detection rate in each year from 2001 to 2007 are: Bihar, Jharkhand, Kerala, Maharashtra and Uttar Pradesh. In all, eight of the 18 states under-performed on detection rate perpetually over the years. This aspects needs to be addressed for the success of the programme.

Bid to involve Political will in Drive Against TB[22]

TB control programmes without political leadership, particularly in India, is likely to plateau and gradually lose its effectiveness with increasing instances of multidrug resistance. Politicians can not absolve themselves of their responsibility of helping control this epidemic. Providing high quality drugs and laboratories through the revised national tuberculosis programme is only partially doing the job of stemming the epidemic. To ensure greater access to treatment and to motivate greater demand, political leadership is required at the constituency level. Need for accountability of the political

[22]The Hindu, New Delhi, March 26, 2009.

Table 4.8: Distribution of states and union territories for which both the detection rate (DR %) and success rate (SR %) are available over a period of seven years from 2001–07, India

	2001		*2002*		*2003*		*2004*		*2005*		*2006*		*2007*	
	DR	**SR**	**DR**	**SR**	**DR**	**SR**	**DR**	**SR**	**DR**	**SR**	**DR**	**SR**	**DR**	**SR**
Period 2001-07														
All areas covered	56	84	59	85	69	87	72	86	66	86	66	86	70	86
Andhra Pradesh	56	84	71	81	81	87	77	86	74	87	74	87	81	87
Assam	73	81	78	86	62	88	70	82	55	80	64	82	74	86
Bihar	37	90	47	92	48	92	49	90	27	89	27	83	45	83
Delhi	79	83	92	84	80	82	81	85	83	87	90	87	87	86
Gujarat	53	78	57	82	66	84	72	85	69	86	77	87	78	87
Haryana	56	79	64	83	57	82	70	83	57	82	60	83	59	85
Himachal Pradesh	61	90	65	90	82	89	82	88	78	89	81	89	81	89
Jharkhand	47	83	59	90	55	93	63	93	50	90	64	87	73	89
Karnataka	61	84	62	82	66	85	65	81	63	82	60	79	61	78
Kerala	60	89	63	89	45	89	45	89	45	87	43	84	64	83
Madhya Pradesh	55	82	54	84	55	85	60	84	53	83	54	83	56	85
Maharashtra	48	84	50	85	59	86	67	87	66	87	65	87	66	86
Manipur	82	87	72	85	77	88	68	85	53	86	59	85	55	85

Contd...

Table 4.8: Distribution of states and union territories for which both the detection rate (DR %) and success rate (SR %) are available over a period of seven years from 2001–07, India (*Contd...*)

	2001		*2002*		*2003*		*2004*		*2005*		*2006*		*2007*	
	DR	**SR**	**DR**	**SR**	**DR**	**SR**	**DR**	**SR**	**DR**	**SR**	**DR**	**SR**	**DR**	**SR**
Orissa	83	88	79	86	91	87	65	84	60	82	59	85	65	86
Rajasthan	69	85	76	86	79	88	81	88	77	88	80	88	81	89
Tamil Nadu	45	79	59	83	73	87	82	88	77	88	68	84	68	83
Uttar Pradesh	67	85	73	90	55	90	54	84	49	87	52	87	56	86
West Bengal	53	84	51	84	64	86	70	87	76	87	78	87	77	87
Period 2002-07														
Punjab	*	*	38	82	41	87	50	85	48	86	55	84	56	85
Period 2003-07														
Arunachal Pradesh	*	*	*	*	91	82	81	87	89	97	105	90	100	87
Chandigarh	*	*	*	*	77	80	76	85	76	89	82	86	75	86
Chhattisgarh	*	*	*	*	47	82	62	85	55	85	59	86	57	87
Nagaland	*	*	*	*	47	87	55	84	53	91	60	87	74	90
Sikkim	*	*	*	*	82	87	125	89	115	88	116	88	112	86
Uttaranchal	*	*	*	*	44	95	61	92	51	87	49	87	61	89

Contd...

Table 4.8: Distribution of states and union territories for which both the detection rate (DR %) and success rate (SR %) are available over a period of seven years from 2001–07, India (*Contd...*)

	2001		*2002*		*2003*		*2004*		*2005*		*2006*		*2007*	
	DR	**SR**	**DR**	**SR**	**DR**	**SR**	**DR**	**SR**	**DR**	**SR**	**DR**	**SR**	**DR**	**SR**
Period 2004-07														
Meghalaya	*	*	*	*	*	*	67	76	50	79	66	81	77	82
Mizoram	*	*	*	*	*	*	82	86	74	86	77	91	95	91
Period 2005-07														
Goa	*	*	*	*	*	*	*	*	53	77	52	70	51	73
Jammu & Kashmir	*	*	*	*	*	*	*	*	25	86	33	83	43	87
Pondicherry	*	*	*	*	*	*	*	*	78	75	85	78	80	91
Tripura	*	*	*	*	*	*	*	*	40	89	49	87	56	90
Period 2006-07														
Andaman & Nicobar					*	*	*	*	*	*	93	82	85	86
D & N Haveli	*	*	*	*	*	*	*	*	*	*	75	78	62	82
Daman & Diu	*	*	*	*	*	*	*	*	*	*	67	93	67	92
Lakshadweep	*	*	*	*	*	*	*	*	*	*	14	100	12	71
Number of areas	18	18	19	19	25	25	27	27	31	31	35	35	35	35

Notes: *Stands for either not covered or incomplete data for calculation.

leadership in controlling tuberculosis has been raised by the Indian Network for People Living with HIV/AIDS which represents the most vulnerable population. The nationwide campaign was organized as a follow-up to the international theme of 2009 World TB Day.

The campaign coincided with the election process in the country and was simultaneously launched from different State capitals. Rallies of tuberculosis patients and grassroots workers were organized to mark the event. During the campaign, grassroots advocacy workers in each Lok Sabha constituency were expected to record the contribution of the related Member of Parliament in controlling TB in her/his constituency. The recording included a set of 18 questions for the MPs. The parameters as developed by the campaign comprised factors including consciousness, communication, campaign, co-operation and capacity-building. The effort would help compile a baseline report card of political leadership for TB control in India.

Bid to involve Civil Society and Others in Drive against TB[23]

As many as 45 civil society organizations from across India converged in the capital to discuss the re-emergence of tuberculosis and work out strategies to counter it. Experts agreed that although much was being said about the success of India's Revised National Tuberculosis Control Programme (RNTCP) to meet global goals, much work still remained to be done.

The representatives resolved to address new emerging challenges at the grassroots level and called for understanding the changing nature of the disease. The efforts made so far by the government and civil society were acknowledged but a need to renew commitments to address emerging challenges and old threats that have resurfaced was felt. The seriousness of the situation may be illustrated by the massive partnership of more than 2,500 NGOs, 260 medical colleges, and 210 corporate houses that enabled the RNTCP to achieve its goal. Despite this success, the experts agreed for the need for close coordination and clear communication among the partners

[23]India bears highest TB burden, The Tribune, New Delhi, November 10, 2008.

particularly to reach those who were currently outside the reach of the public health system.

The recent reports have identified major challenges for the programme that include limited community awareness, suboptimal community participation and sense of ownership, emerging challenges of TB-HIV co-infection requiring accelerated health system response, and limitations in access to quality-TB care for the hard to reach, marginalized and vulnerable populations.

India's priority has to be to educate people at the grassroots. The level of awareness about TB, its symptoms, treatment and prevention, is woefully inadequate even in urban and metropolitan areas. The situation in rural areas is any body's guess.

Management of Drug-resistant TB

The findings of the community-based drug resistance surveillance (DRS) conducted in Gujarat and Maharashtra that the prevalence of drug-resistant TB in new cases was about 3%, raised a concern at the highest level of the Government. This was highlighted in the address of the then minister of Health and Family Welfare, Government of India[24]. The message was that the most effective means of preventing further resistance was through maintaining and improving the quality of treatment and more importantly promoting the rational use of anti-TB drugs.

The national programme, therefore, initiated the DOTS plus services for management of MDR-TB in Gujarat and Maharashtra in early 2007. This facility was scheduled to be extended to other states across the country in a phased manner by 2009-10. Additionally, TB/HIV coordination activities implemented jointly by the RNTCP and National AIDS Control Programme were scaled up to cover 14 states.

A 10-point counseling tool on TB was developed by RNTCP for use by counselors in the Voluntary Counseling and Testing Centers. RNTCP was implementing the 2006 global strategy to prevent TB and reach the TB-related targets of the MDGs by 2015.

---

[24]Drug-resistant TB a major challenge, The Hindu, New Delhi, December 15, 2007.

The challenges to the programme were identified as:

- Sustaining the basis DOTS services for the next several years with systems in place to enhance the quality and reach of the programme.
- Implementation of the programme in states with weak health systems and establishment of a national laboratory network for an accurate diagnosis of MDR.

DOTS Plus

Despite the presence of drug resistant tuberculosis in India virtually since anti-tubercular drugs were introduced, it was only recently that the government launched DOTS Plus programme to take on the challenge of MDR-TB which was more difficult and costly to treat than drug susceptible TB. The programme initiated the DOTS Plus services for management of MDR-TB in the states of Gujarat and Maharashtra in early 2007. Extension of this service for other states was to be completed by 2009–10. Simultaneously, TB/HIV coordination activities implemented jointly by the RNTCP and National AIDS Control Programme were to be scaled up to cover 14 states. Recent work has shown that treatment of MDR-TB is feasible and cost-effective even in settings of very limited resource. When patients default initially or the first category of TB drugs fail to work, there is still the option of treating him or her with CAT II, under the DOTS regimen itself. Defaulting again is what will put the patient at great risk of multidrug resistance.

Since the diagnosis and treatment of MDR-TB cases are complex, RNTCP has developed national guidelines based on the ones given by WHO. Under the DOTS Plus strategy the diagnosis of MDR-TB will be made at the Intermediate Reference Laboratories (IRLs) accredited to perform culture and Drug Sensitivity Testing (DST). After diagnosis, the treatment of MDR-TB patients is assigned to certain DOTS Plus sites, established in tertiary care centres. The CAT IV regimen of treatment, prescribed for MDR-TB, is given daily under DOTS at the centre during a short period of in-patient care. Follow-up action is initiated to deliver the drugs through DOTS again, making it available directly to the patient. At the end of 2008, the DOTS Plus services were available in seven states: Gujarat,

Maharashtra, Andhra Pradesh, Haryana Delhi, Kerala, West Bengal and Tamil Nadu. DOTS Plus services were expected to be available in all States by 2010.

DOTS Plus Programme in Haryana[25]

Haryana after introducing DOTS Plus programme, became the first state in North India and only the third in the country, after Maharashtra and Gujarat, to provide free second line treatment to TB patients who have become multidrug-resistant because of incomplete and inadequate TB treatment. The cost of treatment for multidrug-resistant patients was estimated around Rs.1 lakh per patient which was free of cost under the Revised National TB Control Programme (RNTCP).

In the first phase seven districts—Rohtak, Panipat, Sonepat, Jind, Karnal, Jhajjar and Bhiwani—were to be covered. The second phase was to cover the remaining districts in the State.

Budget and Programme

India, having one-fifth patients of the world, has hiked budget for TB-control programmes from Rs. 740 crores for 2000–2005 to Rs 1,156 crores for October 2005 September 2010. DOTS Programme of India covering 100% of more than 1 billion people was the largest health care programme in the world. Now every district has microscopic and DOTS treatment centers - a microscopy unit for every 1,00,000 people and treatment cells for every 50,000 persons.

[25]The Hindu, New Delhi, October 14, 2008.

Part II

Socioeconomic Aspects: A Case Study of Delhi

5

Background

"Social and economic research is ... needed to enable programmes to take into account the views of their intended beneficiaries,... and to respond to the specific needs of those groups and of communities".

United Nations Population Fund, International Conference on Population and Development, Cairo, 1994

5.1 INTRODUCTION

Tuberculosis and poverty form a vicious circle. It kills more adults than any other infectious disease. More than 80% of the people infected with the disease are in the economically productive years of lives (15–54 years). On the one hand, it decreases a person's capacity to work and on the other, it increases the economic burden due to added expenses on treatment. Generally, poor people seek and receive inadequate health care that often inhibits the detection of TB and thus adds to the seriousness of the impact of the disease. Despite this association, the disease is known to spread across all socio-economic strata. It causes huge economic and social disruption and hampers development of the country. An adult suffering from TB loses 3 to 4 months of working time and over 20–30% of the households annual income. In case of death, income for about 15 years is lost to the family[1].

[1]TB India 2005, RNTCP Status Report, Central TB Division, Directorate General of Health Services, Ministry of Health and Family Welfare, Government of India, New Delhi , p.8–9.

The social burden of TB is also quite heavy, particularly in the case of women. The stigma attached to TB causes damage to men and women differently. While men have to deal with stigma at their work place and the community level, women have to face ostracism within the household and in the immediate neighbourhood. In the case of women, the disease adversely affects the child-care. Children of infected mothers often drop-out of school in order to supplement the family income and to help take care of siblings. The disease can as well cause infertility in the case of infected women[2].

The above findings apparently lack support from large scale studies. Our literature review shows that large scale surveys have rarely been carried out to substantiate the preceeding observations. Most of the interrelationships that have been noted so far are based on the reflections of a cumulative version of small scale studies and experiences of health service providers. During the course of our research we could locate limited number of studies mostly based on localized surveys covering small sample sizes. Although these studies lack extrapolation and generalization, their findings reviewed below provide useful insight in the socio-economic implications of the disease.

5.2 SOCIOECONOMIC IMPACT OF TUBERCULOSIS

A study on the *Socioeconomic Impact of Tuberculosis on Patients and Families in India* by R. Rajeswari, et al (1999)[3] covering both men and women attempted to:

1. Assess the expenditure involved in tuberculosis diagnosis and treatment and its effects on patient's families.
2. Estimate the loss of working hours due to active disease and/or its sequelae and the consequential loss of income.
3. Assess the difference in economic impact due to gender.

Despite the inclusion of the word "India" in the title, the study is very much localized. It covered a small sample of 304

[2]Ibid., p. 9.

[3]*Socio-economic impact of tuberculosis on patients and family in India*, R Rajeswari, R Balasubramanian, M Muniyandi, S Geetharamani, X Thresa, P Venkatesan, Int. J Tuberc Lung Dis 3 (10), 869–877, 1999.

(184 males, 120 females) patients from urban and rural areas and attending government and NGO hospitals/clinics situated in Chennai City and two rural districts of Tamil Nadu. Patients receiving treatment from private practitioners in Chennai City were also included in the sample. Newly detected sputum-positive pulmonary tuberculosis patients receiving short-course chemotherapy were enrolled for the study. Monthly visits were made to each center until required number of patients were interviewed. Patients were chosen at random according to their availability at the clinics. The details of the sample distribution are given in Table 5.1.

Table 5.1: Distribution of sample size by region, type of health facility and gender

Region	*Type of hospital*	*Gender*		
		Male	**Female**	**Person**
Rural	Government	61	40	101
	NGO	37	15	52
	Total (Rural)	98	55	153
Urban	Government	60	41	101
	NGO	14	11	25
	Private	12	13	25
	Total (Urban)	86	65	151
All	Total	184	120	304

At the initial stage of the study, 17 focus group discussions (FGD), each consisting of 8–10 persons (patients, village elders and young men/women), were carried out. These discussions centered around health seeking behaviour in general, with particular reference to respiratory infections, costs involved in diagnosis and treatment, and the impact on the family. These FGDs paved the way to prepare a semi-structured pre-coded interview schedule for the survey.

This pioneering study, well conceived, designed and implemented, despite its limitations on account of coverage and resulting wider applicability, has documented the socio-economic and personal sufferings of tuberculosis patients. Some of the salient findings of the study are given below:

1. A significant number of patients (40–50%), although ultimately diagnosed and treated in government health facilities, were found to have incurred heavy expenditure while seeking a diagnosis in the private sector.
2. Expenditure during treatment was similar among patients attending government and NGO health facilities where anti-TB drugs were provided free of charge. By contrast the cost was 10–15 times higher for private patients. More than two-thirds of patients borrowed money.
3. Non-medical expenditure also imposed a disproportionate burden on poor households.
4. With TB, there is loss of productivity and increase in debts.
5. Most of the work days lost was in the pre-treatment period. Of the average 83 work days lost, 48 and 35 were for pre-treatment and post-treatment periods respectively.
6. Women were more vulnerable to ill-health which affected child survival and family welfare.
7. Fear and stigma associated with TB had a greater impact on women than men.
8. TB had a considerable impact on patients households in terms of income, health, education and nutrition, particularly when the patient was a wage earner. This impact was especially visible in school children, particularly when the patient was a breadwinner.

The study by S Geetha Ramani et al. (2001), on *Socioeconomic Impact of Parental Tuberculosis on Children*[4], attempted to explore the impact of pulmonary tuberculosis in respect of:

1. Social, economic and demographic characteristics of patients who were parents.
2. The child care function of mothers who were patients.
3. Effect on children's education.

The sample consisted of 167 (98 males, 69 females) patients and their 276 (170 male and 106 female) children. The sample

[4]*Socioeconomic Impact of Parental Tuberculosis on Children*, S Geetharamani, M Muniyandi, R Rajeswari, R Balasubramanian, X Theresa and P Venkatasan, Ind. J Tub. 2001, 48, 91.

considered in this study was a sub -sample of the study reported by R Rajeswari et al (1999)[5] and therefore shared similar limitations towards its wider applicability. Findings of the study listed below, despite the limitations, are worth noting.

1. In the case of female patients, as expected, household activities were generally affected adversely but the worst impact of the disease was on child-care. Mother's illness caused a substantial drop in the proper child caring which fell from a level of 64% of mothers giving satisfactory care to their children to 35% in rural areas and from 74 to 33% in urban areas.
2. Mother's illness also affected adversely the education of children. Those who dropped-out of school comprised 11% of the children (8% in rural areas and 13% in urban areas). The drop-out percentage was significantly higher in families with 5 or more members and children living with both parents compared to single parent families. Thirty-four percent of study parents could not buy school-books or adequate food because of loss of income and 20% of the children were obliged to take up jobs in order to supplement family's income. The study, though based on a small sample, clearly showed the adverse impact of parental tuberculosis on their children's education as well as on children's labour. In the views of researchers this was a clear warning which needed to be addressed to prevent prevalent child labour in the country and encourage children to attend and continue in educational institutions.

5.3 TUBERCULOSIS AND WELL-BEING

Tuberculosis often leaves its impact on physical, social and mental state of patients. This was revealed in a study by R Rajeshwari et al. (2005)[6] which explored *the Perception of Tuberculosis Patients about Their Physical, Mental and Social Well-being: A Field Report from South India*. To understand

---

[5]See footnote 3.

[6]*Perceptions of Tuberculosis Patients About Their Physical, Mental And Social Well-Being: A Field Report From South India*, R Rajeswari, M Muniyandi, R Balasubramanian, PR Narayanan, Social Science and Medicine, 60 (2005), 1845–1853.

patients perception of TB and its impact on their lives, 610 (404 males and 206 females) patients who were cured or had completed treatment out of 980 patients registered in 37 government health facilities in Tiruvallur district, Tamil Nadu, were interviewed at two points in time (July and December 2000). Researchers felt that a better understanding of these issues would help in framing an improved design of client-oriented comprehensive TB programme to enhance the quality of life of patients. The study assessed the perception of patients about:

i. Their illness
ii. Their reaction to initial diagnosis; and
iii. The impact of the disease and treatment, on their health (both physical and mental) and social well-being.

Observations on the initial reaction to diagnosis revealed that patients had a poor knowledge of TB, only 12% of male and 16% of female patients were aware of the infectious aetiology of the disease. When diagnosis was disclosed to patients their reactions varied from worry (male 50%, female 58%), suicidal thoughts (male 9%, female 9%) to depression (male 7%, female 10%). Two percent of men and 3% of women thought they would die of TB. Patients who accepted the diagnosis of tuberculosis, when it was disclosed to them, formed a low share of the total at 31% for males and 24% for females. 'Good health status' was perceived initially before the start of the treatment by less than 7% of patients, and compared to the status at the onset of illness, the perception improved significantly to more than 78% after treatment. Despite micro-biological cure, 47% of patients continued to have respiratory symptoms; this was significantly higher among patients who had delayed taking action for more than 3 months. Only 54% of patients perceived 'happy mental status' at the end of treatment, and there was no change in social stigma in both men and women. Authors have drawn attention of the authorities implementing RNTCP to address issues such as continued respiratory symptoms, persistence of stigma, and poor emotional quality of life of patients with tuberculosis, even after they were cured. Additionally, researchers have made a strong case for the Programme to be strengthened by including the provisions for social support, counseling and health education of patients which were considered to improve the rehabilitation of patients to normal life-style after the treatment.

5.4 TUBERCULOSIS AND POVERTY

Tuberculosis has historically been associated with high level of poverty, as it has traditionally been recognized as a disease of the poor. The study linking the disease to poverty[7], based on the review of several studies and reported in ICMR (Indian Council of Medical Research) Bulletin, noted that the intensity of the relationship purely in economic terms originated from:

i. The size of the problem; and
ii. The fact that in developing countries the majority of those affected are in the economically active age-segment of the population.

This review provides evidence of increased prevalence of infection and disease in the low income groups of population compared to middle income groups. People in both of these income groups were also placed most unfavourably compared to higher income groups. The prevalence of infection and disease in the low income group was noted to be about 1.5 times higher than that in middle income groups. The people in higher income groups showed negligible chance of getting the infection or the disease.

The cause and effect relationship between TB and poverty is a matter of debate. No conclusive evidence has been advanced as to which one causes which one. It is true that, since 19th century, many studies carried out in India and elsewhere have suggested that poverty, homelessness, substance abuse, physiological stress, poor nutritional status and crowded living conditions are inextricably linked and all these increase the risk of TB. It is equally true that TB impoverishes families, undermines economic progress, impedes human

[7]Tuberculosis and Poverty, ICMR Bulletin, Vol. 32, No.3, (March, 2002), Division of Publication and Information, ICMR, New Delhi.

development and traps the world's poorest and the most marginalized people in vicious cycle of disease and poverty.

The association between poverty and tuberculosis was also reported by a study on *Tuberculosis Control Programme. Is it pro-poor*? by M Muniyandi et al. (2004)[8]. The objective of the study was to assess whether the TB programme was outreaching the poorer segment of the community. To assess this the researchers interviewed 896 (91%) of the 980 TB patients registered for treatment under government health facilities in the state of Tamil Nadu[9]. The researchers observed that 64% of the patients compared to 51% of the community were having low standard of living. This finding may be interpreted in two ways. One, as noted in the study, it signified that the programme was pro-poor. Two, it may also be interpreted to imply that TB was more prevalent among the poor families. While the former interpretation is conclusive, the latter is debatable. Most of the studies that link poverty and TB are based on the economic profile of patients who are generally registered for treatment with public health service providers. Hardly any study attempts to look at the economic profile of patients attending the private health providers. There appears a need for a large scale study to determine the link between poverty and TB and quantify the relationship.

5.5 FINANCIAL BURDEN OF TUBERCULOSIS ON PATIENTS

Tuberculosis in the presence of poverty causes huge financial burden on patients and their families particularly in India. The assessment of this burden has been the objective of a study by Muniyandi and associates (2005)[10]. The purpose of the study was to estimate the costs incurred by tuberculosis patients treated under RNTCP in Tiruvaller district, Tamil Nadu, where services were decentralized for diagnosis and treatment. In all

[8]Tuberculosis Control Programme – Is it Pro Poor? M Muniyandi, Rajeshwari R, R Balasubramanian, SAARC J TB L Dis and HIV; 2004 (1), 14–19.
[9]For details of this sample see footnote 6.
[10]*Costs to Patients with Tuberculosis Treated under Dots Programme*, M Muniyandi, Rajeswari R. and R. Balasubramanian, Indian J Tuberc 2005; 52: 188–196.

455 patients registered under RNTCP between June and December 2000 were interviewed to collect data on demographic and socio-economic characteristics of patients, expenditure incurred due to illness and effect of illness on employment. The study covered the direct[11] medical and non-medical costs and indirect[12] and total costs[13] incurred on account of tuberculosis before and during treatment. In addition, standard of living index[14] (SLI) for patients was calculated.

Patients of low SLI formed the majority (62%). The direct costs including medical (investigation plus drugs) and travel, lodging, special food and escort expenses during pre-treatment period were more than that during the treatment period. The median costs for the two periods were Rs 340 and 100 respectively. The indirect costs included loss of wages, decreased earning ability and long term disability. More than 50% of patients did not incur any indirect costs in both pre-treatment and during treatment periods and overall total costs were Rs 1,398. About 12% of the patients lost more than 60 workdays. After completion of treatment about 88% returned to work.

This study, according to researchers, for the first time did economic evaluation of DOTS programme and confirmed that, for TB patients, the strategy saved costs, achieved effective cure, saved lives, reduced disability and decreased work absenteeism, especially among the poor, enabling them to return to work at the earliest, thus increasing their productivity.

---

[11]Direct costs include consultation fees and money spent on investigations and drugs (medical expenditure), money spent on travel, lodging, special food and expenditure incurred for persons accompanying the patient were classified as non-medical expenditure.

[12]Indirect costs were classified as loss of wages due to illness, decreased earning ability due to illness, or long term disability that necessitated change in type of work.

[13]Total cost includes the expenditure incurred during pre-treatment as well as during treatment under direct and indirect costs.

[14]The standard of living index was calculated as weighted sum of scores using factors such as type of house, availability and type of toilet facility, main fuel used for cooking, source of drinking water, availability of separate room for cooking, ownership of house, ownership of land, ownership of livestock and ownership of durable goods.

The estimated expenses might be on the lower side because the study covered only out-patients in rural government health facilities. No consideration was given to in-patients as well as those in urban areas.

These estimates of costs may be compared to those given by R Rajeswari et al.[15], for treatment of tuberculosis in the pre-RNTCP period. This comparison shows the advantages of the current programme particularly for the poor population. Rajeswari et al. found that direct mean cost for treatment in the total sample was Rs 2,052 and indirect cost was Rs 3,934. This gives the mean total cost as Rs 5,984. When this cost is compared to a much lower cost estimated by Muniyandi et al. at Rs 1,398, it becomes obvious that RNTCP has the potential to save about Rs. 4,500 or so per TB patient treated.

The distribution of cost incurred by TB patients is highly skewed. This is shown by studies reported by R Rajeswari et al. and Muniyandi et al. For example, while the former study noted that the cost of treatment for TB could vary from Rs 0 to 31,083 per patient, the latter noted the range as 0 to 30,360 for pre-treatment cost and 0 to 13,712 for during treatment cost. This wide range compared to mean or median costs signifies presence of a lot of uncertainty that prevails in diagnosis and treatment costs from patient to patient.

Also, R Rajeswari et al. found that cost of treatment in government health facilities in urban areas was higher than that in rural areas. The respective mean costs were Rs 1,610 and 1,079. By contrast the cost for treatment in urban areas for NGO health facilities were lower than that in rural areas with respective means being Rs 1,408 and 1,840. This contradiction is hard to reconcile.

5.6 KNOWLEDGE, ATTITUDE AND PRACTICE (KAP)

To counter the fear and stigma and promote the discussion about the disease at family/neighbourhood levels, the IEC

[15]See footnote 4.

(Information, Education and Communication) strategy of RNTCP sponsored a study on knowledge, attitude and practice (KAP). The aim of the study was to promote better understanding and its cure, improve the quality of TB patient care (patient-friendly) and to reduce stigma.

The KAP study was conducted by RK Swamy BBDO and Center for Media Studies (CMS) for the Central TB Division (CTD), Ministry of Health and Family Welfare. It was carried out in three phases – baseline, mid-term and end round. The Reports for these rounds are available through the MOHFW[16]. This study concentrated on the assessment changes in knowledge level, behavioural patterns and habits of target audience of beneficiaries, health service providers and influencers/opinion leaders. The specific objectives of study were (parentheses present changes in objectives during mid-term/end-term as underlined where as those only in the end round as italicized).

i. To assess (<u>the change</u>) in awareness level of the beneficiaries, opinion leaders and health service providers regarding Tuberculosis and DOTS (*increase in target groups reached with information that DOTS is the correct treatment, it is available free in patient-wise boxes*).

ii. To understand the (<u>change in</u>) attitude of the three segments towards TB patients with particular reference to gender.

iii. To know (<u>gauge change in</u>) the tuberculosis related practices in the three segments (*respondent groups) (increase in the level of awareness about TB diagnosis and DOTS treatment amongst practitioners*).

iv. To assess the interest of opinion leaders and heath service provides in becoming a part of RNTCP/DOTS programme.

v. To identify the information needs and preferred sources of the beneficiaries for receiving messages related to TB (the sources of information about TB and related issues).

---

[16]These reports are available on the website of the MOHFW http://www.tbcindia.org.

vi. To map the media habits/preferences of the beneficiaries (identify the change in information needs related to TB and preferred sources for the same).

vii. *To identify the increase (if any) in state and district level capacity to plan and execute IEC activities.*

The study was spread over nine states (Himachal Pradesh, Uttar Pradesh in the north, Tamil Nadu, Andhra Pradesh in the south; West Bengal, Manipur replaced by Meghalaya subsequently because of political unrest in the east; and Chhattisgarh, Maharashtra and Gujarat in the west). It covered a sample of two districts per state and a sample per district included 80 (50 urban slums and 30 rural) households, 10 opinion leaders and 12 health service providers. The base line, mid-term and end-round surveys were conducted, respectively, in November 2002, 2004 and September 2005.

The study has documented some interesting facts that reveal the ground realities about the status of knowledge, attitude and practice relevant to RNTCP. Some of these summarized below are encouraging where as others are of concern.

On the positive side it was encouraging to note that:

- Respondents believed that TB was curable and after treatment people could lead a normal life.
- Respondents preferred allopathic system of medicines and government health facilities over other systems and facilities.
- Community and opinion leaders preferred government hospitals over others for diagnosis of the disease and DOTS centre for treatment.
- Opinion leaders and private doctors were keen to become a part of DOTS programme.
- Hospitals were identified as the prime source of information both for the households and for the opinion leaders. This was followed by TV.

Some of the concerns identified by the study were:

- More than half of the opinion leaders were not aware of DOTS and DOTS centres.

- Health service providers and doctors reported that people were reluctant to come forward for treatment or reveal previous incidences of TB in the family. Prevalence of substantial degree of stigma related to the disease was noted as the chief reason.
- A large proportion of respondents believed that talking, sharing dishes with infected person and sharing of clothing and bedding with infected person spreads TB.
- Respondents believed that persons having low immunity and living in congested localities were prone to getting TB infection.

The needs identified by the study include the following:

- Dissemination for information on TB related to prevention and precaution.
- Organization of a comprehensive training programme in the field of IEC and monitoring the influence of the campaign for officers of all levels involved in RNTCP.

In the context of improving the performance of RNTCP it is relevant to know the factors that influence people's action and motivate them to take measures leading to cured/completed treatment, defaulted or even not to avail any treatment. Therefore the findings of the KAP survey, though, important in the context of the activities of the RNTCP, provide limited help for taking action towards improving the performance of the programme and improve the detection and success rates. Consequently there is a need for undertaking a comprehensive study which could address all these issues. Since a satisfied patient is the best advertisement for the success of the performance of the RNTCP, it is important to assess their expectations and ground realities of the situation and develop appropriate strategies to meet or counter them as the case may demand.

6

Tuberculosis in Delhi

6.1 INTRODUCTION

Spread of tuberculosis in Delhi has recently become a matter of concern. According to a recent report it is estimated that, the annual incidence of the disease at 2.4% is close to almost three hundred thousand. This is despite the fact that Delhi is one of the two states where the tuberculosis control programme has been augmented with DOTS+ which takes care of those patients who develop drug resistance. According to the report the cause for concern comes from the fact that the disease is affecting the young and affluent section of the population. It is estimated that those aged 18–35 year olds account for almost 60 percent of TB infections in upscale clinics and hospitals in Delhi[1]. This shows that tuberculosis is no longer only the 'poor man's disease'. A compromised immunity caused by lifestyle factors such as stress and poor diet to keep the weight under control lower the body's immune system and lead to full-blown infection even in the affluent young, who traditionally did not suffer from this disease.

Most of the cases being reported are of "reactivation of latent TB", where prior exposure to infection results in the disease due to various factors, including compromised immunity.

It is not just pulmonary tuberculosis that is on the rise. Other forms like Brain TB, bone TB and gland TB are also rising. It

[1]HT Nation, New Delhi, March 25, 2007.

may be noted that these forms can not be detected by sputum test and/or by X-ray, the two widely used tests done under the tuberculosis control programme. According to doctors the spinal tuberculosis has recently been detected and made rapid inroads in Delhi's affluent people.

TB STALKING THE RICH AND YOUNG

Stress, long work hours, crash diets make them vulnerable

–*HT Nation, New Delhi, March 25, 2007*

6.2 MANAGING TUBERCULOSIS IN DELHI

Under RNTCP, the pilot project started in Delhi in October 1993 with centres at Gulabi Bagh followed by at LRS. It was expanded to include Nehru Nagar and Moti Nagar in 1995/1996. Full coverage was achieved by January 1999.

With an estimated population of 16 million in 2006, the programme in the state of Delhi was implemented through 21 TB Units segmented into six zones. Each TB Unit is comprised of a number of DOTS cum microscopic centers and DOTS centres. In all at the time of this study and according to the list provided to the researchers, the programme in Delhi was being implemented through 151 DOTS-cum-microscopic centres and 203 DOTS centres.

Progress during the Year 2005

- Eight folds increase in number of TB patients treated from 5582 (1997) to an all-time record number of 45,647 (2005).
- The case detection rate for new infectious patients has beeen increased four folds from 20% (1997) to 84% (2005) against the international target of 70%.
- The treatment success rate of all types of TB patients increased 3 folds from 30% (1996) to 90% (2005).
- Ten folds decline in the TB death rate from 25% (1996) to 2.3% (2005), therefore averting 9015 deaths due to TB.
- Four folds increase in DOTS centers from 108 (1999) to 432 (2005) with 50 folds increase in NGO participation from 3 centers (1999) to 144 (2005).

- The RNTCP performance has remained consistently at number one position in all quarterly performance reports in 2005 amongst the larger States and UTs in the country.

6.3 PREVALENCE OF TUBERCULOSIS IN DELHI

Official Sources

The RNTCP in Delhi examined about 955 suspected cases for TB per 100,000 persons in 2005[2]. Of this total, about 16% were serum positive. Both these rates were higher than that for the whole country, with suspects examined at about 526 per 100,000 persons of which 13% were serum-positive. Only four states/union Territories, namely Chandigarh, Daman and Diu, Pondicherry and Sikkim, had higher examination rate for suspected cases than Delhi. The annual total case and new smear-positive case detection rates per 100,000 persons in 2005 for Delhi were 285 and 79 respectively. Only Andaman and Nicobar, Daman and Diu, both small in population size, had higher total detection rate than Delhi; and Andaman and Nicobar, Daman and Diu, Sikkim had higher new serum positive detection rate than Delhi. Both the rates for Delhi were much higher than that for the whole country with comparable rates at 128 and 50. The RNTCP in Delhi showed a success rate for new smear-positive patients at 87%. The states which performed marginally better than Delhi in success rate and also had sizeable patient registration were Rajasthan and Tamil Nadu each with success rate of 88%. Thus the RNTCP programme in Delhi appears to have performed very well.

The performance of RNTCP as measured through DR and SR in subsequent years appears to have remained somewhat stable at the rates that prevailed in 2005. For example, the Programme in Delhi examined about 227 suspected cases per 100,000 persons per quarter in 2008, which when annualized matches with the figure at 955 for 2005. The percentage of smear positive cases among the suspected ones remained at 16%, the same as that for 2005. Annual total case detection rate and annual new smear positive case detection rates at 290 and 82

[2]TB India 2006, RNTCP Status Report, op., cit., p. 51–52.

in 2008 were negligibly higher than those at 285 and 79 respectively in 2005. Even the DR and SR in 2008 at 86 and 87 per cent were comparable to those at 83 and 87 in 2005. All the above rates for 2008 were, no doubt, substantially higher than those for all the areas of the country reporting in the years. The comparable figures were: 149, 13; 132, 54 and 72, 87 respectively.

The official statistics since 2005 gives data on quarterly basis for suspected cases examined. RNTCP in Delhi examined 244, 236 and 227 cases per 100,000 persons in 2006, 2007 and 2008 respectively. The comparable rates for the entire country were 140, 143 and 149.

Survey Data

Some idea of the prevalence of tuberculosis in Delhi may be obtained from data given by the NFHS-2 and NFHS-3 presented in Table 6.1. The overall prevalence of tuberculosis in Delhi in 1999 was as high as 511 per 100,000 usual household residents and was very close to the national level at 544. It was also substantially higher than that given by NFHS-1 for the year 1992–93 at 190 and by NFHS-3 at 240 per 100,000 persons per year. Males showed higher prevalence rate compared to females (559 and 459 in 1999; 255 and 221 in 2005–06 respectively). There was clear indication that the prevalence rate increased rapidly with age. The relative levels were in the ratio of about 1:3:5 for children (<15 years), economically active (15–59 years) and the senior (60+ years) age groups of persons. The lowest and highest rates were 189 and 1011. The ratio widened by 2005–06 and it increased to 1:4:8 for the relevant age segments with rates at 71, 278 and 598. The widening of the gap appears to have arisen from the fact that the decline in the prevalence of tuberculosis was progressively slower with rise in age groups.

Urban rural differential in prevalence rate of tuberculosis showed some surprising results. The prevalence was higher in urban than in rural areas. The differential in 1999 was of the order of 5 to one (548 and 92). The differential narrowed substantially to 1.4 to one. It is apparent that RNTCP succeeded more in urban areas but deteriorated in rural areas.

Table 6.1: Number of persons per 100,000 usual household residents suffering from tuberculosis by selected background characteristics, Delhi, 1999 and 2005–06

Background characteristics	*Number of persons per 100,100 suffering from tuberculosis*			
	Tuberculosis reported		*Medically treated tuberculosis*	
	1999	2005–06	1999	2005–06
Age				
Less than 15	189	71	168	71
15–59	629	278	542	265
60+	1,011	598	1,011	598
Sex				
Male	559	255	496	240
Female	459	221	402	221
Residence				
Urban	548	245	483	236
Rural	92	181	92	181
Total	511	240	451	231

Source: National Family Health Survey, India, Delhi, 1998–99 and 2005–06, International Institute for Population Sciences, Mumbai, March 2002, February 2009.

The level and differentials shown by medically treated tuberculosis, which was included in overall tuberculosis, were somewhat similar in nature with lower rates. In 1999, the prevalence of medically treated tuberculosis at 451 was about 60 points less than prevalence of overall tuberculosis. By contrast, the comparative figures for 2005–06 were 231 and 240. The closeness of the differential in 2005–06 between overall and medically treated tuberculosis as compared to that in 1999 might signify the fact that more and more cases were being captured by the TB control programme in recent years. This is good sign as far as control of tuberculosis is concerned. It may safely be assumed, as in NFHS reports, that data on medically treated tuberculosis were expected to present a more reliable measure of prevalence of disease in active stage than the measure based on all reported cases. As expected these rates are somewhat lower than the previously given rates based on all reported cases. However, the differentials shown by rates for medically treated tuberculosis are very similar to that given by rates for all the reported cases.

6.4 KNOWLEDGE AND ATTITUDE TOWARD TUBERCULOSIS

Data on knowledge and attitude toward tuberculosis was collected in NFHS-3. It covers percentage of women and men age 15–49 who had heard of tuberculosis and among those who had heard of TB, percentage with specific knowledge and beliefs, according to background characteristics, in Delhi in 2005–06. Though restricted to a limited age range, the data do show some interesting results as far as knowledge and attitude related to tuberculosis is concerned. The good thing is that almost all respondents have heard of tuberculosis (98% of women and 99% of men). However, among those who had heard of tuberculosis, some matters of concern might be noted. Among such persons, despite almost universal knowledge, only about three-quarters were aware that tuberculosis spreads through the air by coughing or sneezing (76% of women and 79% of men). Further, 78% of women and 69% of men had misconceptions about the spread of tuberculosis. It was encouraging to note that almost all women and men knew that tuberculosis could be cured (96% of women and 97% of men). The stigma attached to tuberculosis could still be seen as 15% of women and 8 percent of men preferred to keep it secret from the neighbours if any member of the family suffered from tuberculosis.

The available data also provide some idea of the differential prevailing in the attitude toward tuberculosis by selected characteristics. Table 6.2, adopted from NFHS shows them in detail. However, some salient points might be worth noting. Of the six characteristics (age, residence, education, religion, caste/tribe and wealth) considered, none showed universality of the differential. Awareness about TB appeared to be marginally associated with level of education only in the case of women where percentage of women who had heard of TB varied from about 94 for of women with 'no education' to almost 100 for those who had 10 or more years of completed education. Women respondents also exhibited some differential in awareness by caste/tribe as well as wealth index. Women belonging to tribal group and also those belonging to poorer groups were less aware of TB than others.

Table 6.2: Percentage of women and men age 15–49 who have heard of tuberculosis (TB), among those who have heard of TB, percentage with specific knowledge and belief, according to background characteristics, Delhi, 2005–06

Backgroud characteristic	*Percentage who have heard of TB*		*Percentage among those who have heard*							
			Reported that TB is spread through the air by coughing or sneezing		*Have misconceptions about transmission of TB*		*Belief that TB can be cured*		*Would want a family member's TB kept secret from the neighbours*	
	Women	*Men*	*Women*	*Men*	*Women*	*Men*	*Women*	*Men*	*Women*	*Men*
Age										
15–19	97.9	98.1	76.5	71.6	77.4	60.0	94.7	97.5	18.0	9.5
20–34	97.9	99.8	75.6	80.5	78.0	69.0	95.0	96.4	15.2	7.7
35–49	98.1	99.1	76.9	83.1	79.5	75.6	96.7	98.7	14.4	7.4
Residence										
Urban	98.1	99.5	76.6	79.9	78.6	69.5	95.6	97.3	15.4	8.1
Rural	97.1	95.7	71.2	73.9	76.3	63.6	94.1	97.7	15.3	5.7
Education										
No education	94.1	97.9	65.1	67.4	69.2	58.7	90.3	89.8	15.3	17.1
<5 yrs completed	96.1	(98.4)	57.8	(65.7)	62.4	(62.4)	92.4	(100.0)	21.9	(14.7)
5-9 yrs completed	98.3	98.6	74.8	74.7	74.2	65.0	95.1	97.1	15.9	7.6
10 or more yrs	99.5	99.9	81.6	84.7	84.1	73.3	97.8	98.6	15.1	6.3
Religion										
Hindu	98.0	99.3	75.8	79.0	78.3	70.0	95.3	97.2	16.1	8.3
Muslim	98.1	98.6	80.4	81.0	82.6	63.7	96.4	97.7	7.3	7.1

Contd...

Table 6.2: Percentage of women and men age 15–49 who have heard of tuberculosis (TB), among those who have heard of TB, percentage with specific knowledge and belief, according to background characteristics, Delhi, 2005–06 (*Contd...*)

Backgroud characteristic	*Percentage who have heard of TB*		*Percentage among those who have heard*							
			Reported that TB is spread through the air by coughing or sneezing		*Have misconceptions about transmission of TB*		*Belief that TB can be cured*		*Would want a family member's TB kept secret from the neighbours*	
	Women	*Men*	*Women*	*Men*	*Women*	*Men*	*Women*	*Men*	*Women*	*Men*
Sikh	99.0	(100)	76.5	(83.7)	68.4	(67.4)	96.9	(100.0)	16.3	(7.0)
Others	96.1	*	70.6	*	80.4	*	98.0	*	22.4	*
Caste/Tribe										
Scheduled caste	96.3	98.8	70.1	72.8	72.7	68.0	93.2	94.0	18.6	9.0
Scheduled tribe	91.2	*	(69.9)	*	(59.7)	*	(96.0)	*	(13.6)	*
Other backward class	96.9	98.5	71.9	78.2	78.0	65.7	92.8	98.2	16.4	9.6
Other	98.8	99.5	78.6	82.0	80.3	69.9	96.6	98.3	14.5	7.2
Wealth Index										
Lowest	*	*	*	*	*	*	*	*	*	*
Second	95.2	98.7	60.2	60.0	60.1	68.6	84.0	94.0	19.3	15.3
Middle	93.0	96.2	66.2	70.7	63.1	61.0	88.0	94.7	22.5	14.3
Fourth	97.2	98.9	69.2	76.1	69.4	66.2	92.1	95.8	13.1	12.3
Highest	98.7	99.7	78.9	82.2	82.1	70.8	97.2	98.2	15.3	5.6
Total	98.0	99.2	76.2	79.4	78.4	69.0	95.5	97.3	15.4	8.0

Note: ( ) based on 25–49 unweighted cases. * Percentage based on fewer than 25 unweighted cases.
Source: National Family Health Survey (NFHS-3) India, 2005-06, Delhi, Table 64.

Further, some interesting differentials are presented by selected characteristics for women and men who had heard of TB. Despite the extensive efforts put in the publicity, only 7–8 women or men for every ten of the respective gender reported that TB could spread 'through the air by coughing and sneezing'. With the exception of age, other five characteristics (residence, education, religion, caste/tribe and wealth index) considered showed substantial differentials. Persons living in rural areas, having lower number of years of education, belonging to other religions, caste/tribe/other backward classes and lower wealth index were relatively fewer in percentage share than those having other characteristic. More women (78%) than men (69%) had misconceptions about transmission of TB. It is somewhat disturbing to note that misconception about transmission of TB is positively linked with number of years of schooling, persons belonging to sikh religion compared to others and wealth index. Better off persons were reported to have misconception more frequently than those not so well off.

The data on 'would want a family's member's TB kept secret from the neighbours' provide some differentials that required attention. Overall about 15% of women and 8% of men preferred to keep a family's member's TB secret from neighbours. The prevalence of attitude toward keeping the TB of family's member secret was more frequent among younger, less educated, persons of other religions and of middle and lower wealth index.

Vulnerable Population[3]

Nearly six million of 15 million of Delhi's population is vulnerable to tuberculosis. This is because at least 40% of the population is vulnerable to TB. This number does not mean that there are six million TB patients in Delhi. However, if the population does not take precautions many may fall victim to the disease.

Last financial year nearly 50,000 new cases were put under TB treatment of which 13,695 were sputum infectious cases. The majority of TB victims in Delhi or any other part of the country are migrant labourers, slum dwellers, resident of

[3]The Tribune, New Delhi, September 8, 2008.

crowded localities, and pockets of urban slums. Poor living conditions, malnutrition are other reasons for the spread of the disease.

Since 1997 (till March 2008) 354,116 patients have been put on DOTS regime. This programme has so far saved over 62,000 lives. The death rate has been consistently below 2.5%.

While the general risk of infection is 1.9%, in urban slums it is 2.2%.

Delhi has so far established 188 diagnostic facilities and there are nearly 580 DOTS centers across the city.

Delhi along with Maharashtra and Gujarat has introduced DOTS plus to battle drug resistant TB.

6.5 PERFORMANCE OF DOTS SERVICE IN DELHI

Section 4.3b examined the performance of RNTCP in different states/union territories of India. Two parameters considered for the purpose are detection rate for new-smear-positive TB cases (DR) and success rate for cure/completion of treatment (SR) among those registered. We extend this concept to examine the performance of DOTS in different parts of Delhi. Like before, we use the data from RNTCP Status Reports issued by the Central TB Division. The data cover the values of DR and SR for twenty reporting units over a period of five years from 2004 to 2008. Table 6.3 presents the distribution of reporting units implementing DOTS Programme by performance status, 2004–08, in Delhi.

Although Delhi as a whole met the target criteria for both the DR and SR in all the years considered here, the reporting units showed considerable variability, particularly in the case of DR. Over the period studied DRs varied wildly from 133 (43 for NDMC to 176 for Karawal Nagar) in 2006 to 70 (55 for Gulabi Bagh to 125 for SGM Chest Clinic). It is encouraging to note that the range which was rising from 105 in 2004 to 133 in 2006 with 122 in 2005 registered a downward trend reaching 107 in 2007 and 70 in 2008. By comparison, the range for SR varied within a narrow range of about 10 units from around 81 to 91. It may be observed that more than one-half of the reporting units in 2005, 2006 and 2008 succeeded in meeting

Table 6.3: Distribution of reporting units implementing DOTS programme by performance status 2004–08, Delhi

	2004			*2005*			*2006*			*2007*			*2008*	
	DR	*SR*		*DR*	*SR*		*DR*	*SR*		*DR*	*SR*		*DR*	*SR*
Reporting units with performance below target for detection rate (DR) as well as for success rate (SR)														
Nehru Nagar	58	80										Gulabi Bagh	55	84
Moti Nagar	59	80												
Jhandewalan	69	84												
Reporting units with performance below target for detection rate (DR) but not for success rate (SR)														
NDMC	64	86	Moti Nagar	57	85	RTRM Chest Clinic	48	87	Gulabi Bagh	58	85	LN Chest Clinic	62	87
LRS	68	87	NDMC	43	86	Gulabi Bagh	53	88	NDMC	51	88	LRS	61	89
RK Mission	63	89	Narela	58	87	LN Chest Clinic	60	88	RTRM Chest Clinic	60	88	NDMC	59	91
Gulabi Bagh	48	90	Gulabi Bagh	53	88	NDMC	43	92	LN Chest Clinic	65	88			
LN Chest Clinic	45	92	RTRM Chest Clinic	46	89									
			LN Chest Clinic	45	91									
Reporting units meeting target for detection rate (DR) but not for success rate (SR)														
									Shahadra	139	80	Hedgewar C Clinic	74	83
GTB Chest Clinic	70	81	Shahadra	121	83	Patparganj	127	82	GTB Chest Clinic	107	82	Moti Nagar	84	83

Contd...

Table 6.3: Distribution of reporting units implementing DOTS programme by performance status 2004–08, Delhi (*Contd...*)

	2004			*2005*			*2006*			*2007*			*2008*	
	DR	*SR*		*DR*	*SR*		*DR*	*SR*		*DR*	*SR*		*DR*	*SR*
Karawal Nagar	131	81	Nehru Nagar	79	84	Hedgewar C Clinic	150	84	Moti Nagar	73	83	GTB Chest Clinic	102	84
Patparganj	98	83							Jhandewalan	94	83	Shahadra	132	84
Shahadra	91	84							Nehru Nagar	112	83			
									Karawal Nagar	144	83			
									Narela	81	84			
									Hedgewar C Clinic	88	84			
Reporting units meeting target for detection rate (DR) as well as success rate (SR)														
Narela	77	85	Patparganj	135	86	Jhandewalan	75	85	DDU Chest Clinic	71	86	DDU Chest Clinic	73	85
DDU Chest Clinic	130	85	Jhandewalan	78	87	Nehru Nagar	82	85	SPM Marg	73	86	Jhandewalan	93	85
Kingsway	80	88	GTB Chest Clinic	89	87	Shahadra	114	85	Kingsway	120	86	Nehru Nagar	113	85
SGM Chest Clinic	150	88	Karawal Nagar	165	87	Narela	78	86	Patparganj	127	87	SPM Marg	73	86
SPM Marg	78	89	DDU Chest Clinic	74	88	DDU Chest Clinic	86	86	SGM Chest Clinic	158	87	Karawal Nagar	117	86
BJRM Chest Clinic	92	89	Kingsway	88	88	Karawal Nagar	176	86	LRS	81	88	Kingsway	119	86

Contd...

Table 6.3: Distribution of reporting units implementing DOTS programme by performance status 2004–08, Delhi (*Contd...*)

	2004			*2005*			*2006*			*2007*			*2008*	
	DR	*SR*		*DR*	*SR*		*DR*	*SR*		*DR*	*SR*		*DR*	*SR*
RTRM Chest Clinic	102	91	LRS	91	88	Moti Nagar	73	87	BJRM Chest Clinic	88	90	Narela	84	88
Hedgewar C Clinic	76	*	BJRM Chest Clinic	99	88	SPM Marg	82	87	RK Mission	110	90	RK Mission	97	88
			SPM Marg	72	89	Kingsway	109	87				SGM Chest Clinic	125	88
			RK Mission	90	89	SGM Chest Clinic	115	88				Patparganj	123	89
			SGM Chest Clinic	96	89	GTB Chest Clinic	105	89				RTRM Chest Clinic	73	91
			Hedgewar C Clinic	125	90	LRS	90	90				BJRM Chest Clinic	84	92
						BJRM Chest Clinic	89	91						
						RK Mission	93	91						

the targets for both DR and SR with respective numbers as 12, 14 and 12. For the remaining two years 2004 and 2006 only 8 of the 20 reporting units could be in this group. It was quite encouraging to note that whereas in 2004 almost one-half of the reporting units (9 of 20) failed to meet the target for DR, in subsequent years the number declined and remained at 4 in the years 2006 through 2008. Of the five year period that we have considered, 2007 appears to be less satisfactory than other years as far as meeting the target for SR is concerned. As many as 8 of the 20 reporting units could not meet the target set for SR.

Five consistent target achievers for DR and SR over the entire period of five years were DDU Chest Clinic, Kingsway, SGM Chest Clinic, SPM Marg and BJRM Chest Clinic. The next consistent center was RK Mission which achieved the target over four years from 2005 to 2008. It was surprising to note that LRS could achieve the target on both grounds only in three of the five years. It could not achieve the target for DR in 2004 and 2008. On the negative side three centers, namely NDMC, Gulabi Bagh and LN Chest Clinic, consistently failed to achieve the target for DR. Other centers showed a mixed performance pattern.

7

Methods, Material and Sample Profile

"Valid, reliable, timely, culturally relevant and internationally comparable data form the basis for policy and programme development, implementation, monitoring and evaluation".

United Nations Population Fund, International Conference on Population and Development, Cairo, 1994.

METHODS AND MATERIAL

7.1 INTRODUCTION

The Revised National TB Control Programme (RNTCP), as already mentioned earlier, has set itself a target of achieving new smear-positive case detection and cure rates to the extent of 70 and 85 percent respectively. The Programme, to control prevalence and incidence of tuberculosis in the country, is undergoing a paradigm shift. The success of programme, however, depends upon the productive interaction of its two components: (i) availability of effective and efficient services and (ii) the cooperation of and acceptance by those who are likely to use these services. For successful implementation, it is imperative to have adequate data base that deals with the status of these two components.

Background to the study presented in Chapter 5 showed that tuberculosis, commonly known as poor man's disease, had serious socio-economic implications and was a hindrance to development of the country. In such a situation the co-operation of the users was vital for reduction in prevalence and incidence rates of TB and thereby for success of RNTCP. Our existing knowledge about the socio-economic implications of TB in India was largely based on small and localized sample studies conducted mostly in the state of Tamil Nadu[1]. These studies covered only the TB patients who were under treatment at the time of the survey and any wider applicability of findings could be a matter of debate. The segments of patients identified hereunder were equally important for understanding the socio-economic and psychological implication of the disease but were barely covered.

i. The patients who were cured or completed the treatment some time ago.
ii. The patients who defaulted on the treatment.
iii. Potential or suspected patients who failed to take required action but apparently showed the symptoms generally advertised for people to look for and take appropriate action to contact the health service providers for check-up.

For successful and effective implementation of RNTCP, it will, therefore, be important to assess the socio-economic implications of the disease in a holistic manner and design the programme to counter the negative aspects. In view of our limited knowledge in this field, a study of the profile of TB patients and the socio-economic implications of the disease on patients and their families in the northern part of the country was considered imperative. The present study covering the entire state of Delhi, and sponsored by the Central TB Division of the Directorate General of Health Services, Ministry of Health and Family Welfare, Government of India, was an attempt to fill this gap. To do this a fairly large size sample spread over considerable area was contemplated.

DOTS strategy adopted under RNTCP addresses the issues related to service providers, one of the two elements identified earlier for the successful implementation of the Programme.

[1]Refer to Chapter 5.

The strategy rests on a curative treatment plan for tuberculosis control and is implemented through very productive, effective and efficient interaction of the following five elements.

i. Strong Political and Administrative Commitment.
ii. Availability of quality microscopy services to detect the infectious cases among people attending health care facilities with symptoms of pulmonary tuberculosis, most importantly cough of 3 weeks duration or more.
iii. Regular, dependable and uninterrupted supply of quality anti-TB drugs throughout the health system.
iv. Counseling and swallowing of each dose of medicines under observation of a health or social workers.
v. Monitoring and accountability system for programme supervision and evaluation of treatment of each patient diagnosed.

If any of these five elements is inadequately handled, our ability to consistently cure TB patients is likely to slip through our fingers. At the time of the present study the programme had almost completed the expansion and was poised to enter the maintenance phase. To achieve success at the maintenance stage, it will be essential to ensure the cooperation of the service providers and service users. The present study is an attempt to understanding the mechanics of socio-economic interactions and providing guidelines to successfully combat the disease. Since the TB control programme has only now taken off the ground during the last few years, it will be useful to support it with findings from studies which throw light on the issues and problems emerging under the new dispensation. Studies undertaken during the nineties have little relevance today.

7.2 OBJECTIVES

The primary objective of the study is to assess the socio-economic impact of TB on patients and their families. The secondary objectives will be to study:

1. Socio, demographic and economic differential of TB patients.
2. Reasons for TB patients for not availing services.
3. Reasons for default.
4. Suggestions for reducing the adverse socio-economic impact of TB on patients and their families.

7.3 TIME FRAME

The time period of the study was segmented into (i) preparatory work (three months), (ii) field work, data collection and processing (thirteen months), and data analysis and report writing (four months). The details of the activities carried out under each segment are given below.

Preparatory work included the following:

- Formation of the Technical Advisory Committee (TAC)[2].
- Consultation with researchers/authorities directly/indirectly concerned with the subject[3].
- Recruitment and training of field staff.
- Production of survey instruments including drafting, field testing, finalization in consultation with TAC and CTD, MOHFW, revision and printing.
- Documentation of service providers.
- Visit to selected service providers, establishing rapport, preparing the frame and drawing the sample for the first round of field work, targeting patients who completed treatment/defaulted during the 12/24 months prior to start of the field work.
- Development of software/computer programme for data processing and analysis.

Field work, data collection and processing comprised the following stages:

- Visiting the sampled service providers, establishing rapport and filling the necessary questionnaires.
- Locating the eligible respondents and visiting sample families at their residence and filling up the questionnaire.
- Identifying the suspected cases but not availing the needed health services by snow balling technique and filling questionnaire.
- Visiting default cases, filling up the questionnaire and counseling.

---

[2]Refer to section 7.4.5 below for details.

[3]Dr LS Chauhan, Deputy Director General (TB), Central TB Division, MOHFW, New Delhi.

RP Vashisht, TB Officer, Delhi State.

- Identifying eligible neighbourhood households, visiting them and filling up the questionnaire.
- Visiting the selected service providers and sampling the current patients and filling the exit questionnaires.
- Revisits to patients and their areas of residence.
- Data Screening/Cleaning/Processing (to ensure the quality of data to acceptable level these activities including entry, cleaning and preliminary processing were carried out along with field work).

Data Analysis and Report Writing

The SPSS statistical package was used for data analysis.

7.4 METHODOLOGY

The study uses the sample survey approach to collect data relevant to its objectives. A multi-stage random sample using pps (probability proportional to size) method of selection was utilized. Various aspects of methodology detailed below were finalized in consultation with the TAC and the sponsors. The issue of selecting the sample and sampling methodology was

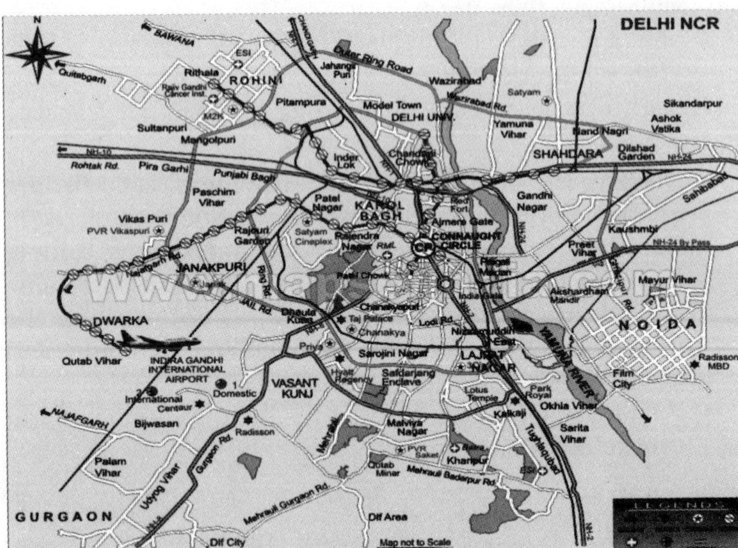

Map of Delhi

discussed at length at the first meeting of the TAC and subsequently at the CTD. On the advice of the TAC, the study took cognizance of the fact that under the RNTCP all the records of the TB patients were kept at the TB unit (TU) level. Each TU comprises a number of DOTS cum microscopic centers and DOTS Centers. Therefore, TU and not service provider as originally planned was made the basis for sampling. Twenty one TUs in the state of Delhi were distributed over six zones; namely, northern, southern, eastern, western, central and old Delhi (Map), were selected for the study.

The present study, to balance the spatial distribution of number of DOTS centers by zone, merged the centers in Old Delhi zone along with those in central zone.

7.4.1 The Study Universe

The study universe consisted of two components. These were: service providers and service users. Each was defined separately for sampling. The *service providers*, categorized in six groups listed below, were considered the lead variable for the study. A service provider eligible for the study was an implementing set-up unit such as a DOTS centre or any other centre including that of a medical practitioner having a distinct clinic for dispensing services for treatment of tuberculosis and qualified to be counted as a service provider for this study. Various types of service providers considered were:

1. DOTS Centers providing service during normal working hours.
2. DOTS Centers supported by NGO(s) where medicines were administered during off hours by specially designated social workers.
3. Dispensaries run and supported by the NGOs.
4. Government Hospitals.
5. Private Hospitals.
6. Private practitioners.

The universe of current and potential *service users* was segmented into the following categories.

1. Patients who were cured or completed the treatment.
2. Patients who had defaulted.

3. Patients who were registered and were currently receiving TB treatment.
4. Patients suspected of TB but not availing RNTCP services.
5. Households in the neighbourhood[4].

Definition of service users adopted in the study: The study uses the following definitions:

Cured: As identified by the service provider from where the sample was selected. A cured case was one which was initially smear-positive, completed treatment and had negative sputum smears, on at least two occasions, one of which was at the completion of treatment.

Treatment completed: A sputum smear-positive patient who had completed treatment, with negative smear at the end of the initial phase but none at the end of treatment, or a sputum smear-negative TB patient who had received a full course of treatment and had not become smear-positive during or at the end of treatment, or an extra-pulmonary TB patient who had received a full course of treatment and had not become smear-positive during or at the end of treatment.

Default: A patient who, at any time after registration, had not taken anti-TB drugs for 2 or more consecutive months.

Currently registered: The registered patients present in the premises of the service provider for receiving their medicines on the day(s) when the exit interview was held.

Suspected TB patients: Persons who satisfied the criteria used by health authorities to advise people to visit the nearest DOTS facility for check-up.

Universe of service providers: All the DOTS centres and private clinics offering treatment for TB defined the universe of service providers.

Universe of service users: The universe of cured and treatment completed patients was defined by all such cases belonging to a period of 12-months prior to the time of field work and related to the particular service provider. In case of

[4]To assess the differential between the socio-economic conditions of households with and without a TB patient, the study covered the households without TB patients in the neighbourhood of the patients in the first two categories.

defaulters, because of the non availability of sufficient number of cases, the period was lengthened to 24-months. In the case of current patients the list obtaining at the time of field work was taken to represent the universe for the particular service provider. No universe was defined for suspected cases as well as for neighbourhood households.

7.4.2 Sample Size and Sampling

Sample Size

To give representation to various areas and type of respondents the following sample size for different categories was adopted.

Category of respondents	*Total*	*Per service provider*
Service Providers	100	1
Service Users – Cured or Completed Treatment	2,500	25
– Defaulted on treatment	500	5
– Currently registered and taking treatment	2,500	25
– Suspected but not availing any treatment	500	5
– Neighbourhood households without TB patient	1,000	10

Sample Allocation

Consistent with the needs of and in consultation with the sponsors, the study placed major emphasis on provision of services through DOTS centers. Therefore, of the 100 service providers in the sample, the study considered 90 DOTS centers and 10 other service providers. The remaining categories of respondents in the sample were split proportionately to conform to this division of service providers. To balance the representation from each zone equally likely, the master sample of service providers was allocated equally to different zones. This procedure was adopted for each category of respondents. Since the DOTS centers formed the major component of the implementation of RNTCP strategy, their heavy representation in the sample was considered important for the programme.

Therefore, the total sample of 100 service providers was split into 90 from DOTS centers and 10 from private practitioners in the vicinity of selected DOTS centers, under the Public Private Partnership (PPP) programme.

From each of the five zones defined earlier, 18 DOTS centers were selected. However, these 18 DOTS centers were allocated to different TUs in the zone in such a way that the number of centers and variability in the TU were taken into account. The allocations of the DOTS centers and total sample by zone are summarized in Table 7.1. The details of the allocation of DOTS centers to different TUs are given in Appendix Table 7.1.

Sampling Frame

The list of DOTS centers (without and/or with NGO collaboration), together with complete address and contact information in Delhi maintained by the Central TB Division provided the frame for lead sampling. This list classified by TB Unit and Zone of its location provided the frame for sampling of DOTS centers.

The frame for the remaining four categories of service providers was prepared with reference to the sampled DOTS centers. This was necessitated by the fact that the available list of DOTS centers served as a useful and cost effective mechanism for preparing the initial sampling frame. Restricting the selection of other service providers to the area of selected DOTS centers was considered a convenient format to capture patients from socio-economic environment that served as the catchment area for the selected DOTS centers.

The sampling frame for various categories of respondents was defined separately in each case depending upon the requirement. The frame for patients who were cured or completed the treatment was prepared from the records at the TUs for a period of 12 months prior to the survey. In the case of patients who defaulted, the period had to be extended to 24 months in some cases to get the required number of responses as stipulated in the survey design. The register of patients kept at the selected DOTS centers provided the frame for conducting exit interviews of current patients. No prior frame was prepared

Table 7.1: Distribution of TUs and sample allocation of DOTS centers and respondents by zones, Delhi , 2005

Zone				Number of Patients				
	*TU**	*DM/DC**	*Number of DC in sample*	*Completed treatment*	*Defaulted*	*Exit interview*	*Suspected but not availing RNTCP services*	*Neighbourhood household without TB patients*
(1)	**(2)**	**(3)**	**(4)**	**(5)**	**(6)**	**(7)**	**(8)**	**(9)**
West	4	71	18	450	90	450	90	180
North	5	94	18	450	90	450	90	180
East	5	82	18	450	90	450	90	180
South	2	59	18	450	90	450	90	180
Central and Old Delhi	5	48	18	450	90	450	90	180
Subtotal	21	354	90	2,250	450	2250	450	900
Others**	NA	NA	10	250	50	250	50	100
Total		**NA**	**100**	**2,500**	**500**	**2500**	**500**	**1,000**

*TU = TB Unit, DM = DOTS Cum Microscopic Center, DC = DOTS Centre.
**Specialist Hospitals and Public/Private Service Providers.
NA Not available.

for capturing the suspected patients as well as the neighbourhood households. The sampling design was prepared accordingly as below.

Sampling

The selection of DOTS centre within a TU was done following a systematic random method. The list of selected DOTS centers by zone and TU in Delhi is given in Appendix Table 7.2.

The selection of cured/treatment completed and defaulted patients was done randomly using systematic sampling procedure. Additional sample was drawn for substitution, in case any of the sampled cured/treatment completed or defaulted person could not be traced at the given address. For exit interview, sampling on the day of interview was done using the systematic method randomly from among the patients attending the centre on that day.

On the basis of information given at the Technical Advisory Committee's meeting it was noted that many patients go to bigger government hospitals not under TUs for treatment of TB. Therefore such places were also considered for sampling particularly for exit interview along with other private service providers. Here the allocation and distribution of the sample was all purposive to extract maximum possible information useful for the study.

In the colonies covered by selected DOTS centers where patients who completed the treatment or defaulted were interviewed, snowballing technique was used to draw the needed sample to get information on persons having symptoms of tuberculosis as per the RNTCP guidelines. The technique was continued till the sample of required size was covered for each selected colony.

Neighbourhood households without TB patients were selected purposively to match the socio-economic characteristics of households which had a patient who was cured or completed the treatment. Selection of suspected cases as well as that of neighbourhood households was done with reference to patients who were cured or completed the treatment and were interviewed in the sample.

7.4.3 Study Tools

The study canvassed six questionnaires, one each for six different respondent categories of target population. These relate to:

1. Service providers
2. Patients who had completed treatment.
3. Patients who had defaulted.
4. Exit schedule for patients (who were registered and were present for receiving medicines on the day of field visit).
5. Suspected TB patients but not availing RNTCP services.
6. Neighbourhood households without TB patients.

7.4.4 Pilot Testing

The initial drafts of the survey questionnaires were pilot tested by the field team recruited and trained for the purpose. The results of the field testing were analyzed and discussed at the first meeting of the TAC. The Committee made a number of significant observations and suggested amendments which were taken care of at the time of finalization of the questionnaires. The revised questionnaires were subsequently discussed in a meeting at the CTD. The questionnaires thus scrutinized and amended were printed and administered to collect field data.

7.4.5 Technical Advisory Committee (TAC)

The study team received guidance from TAC at various stages. This helped in the conduct of the survey in a scientific manner and in developing the modus operandi for such a pioneering study. The input from this committee as well as from the Central TB Division was considered crucial for the success of the study as it was planned to assist the RNTCP to further improve its performance. The assistance of the committee particularly at the initial stages of the planning of the study was extremely useful. The following served as the member of this committee[5].

[5]On suggestion from CTD, the Project co-opted members from time to time who were involved in various activities of the RNTCP. These co-opted members were consulted on ad-hoc basis for specific activities.

1. Dr. Padam Singh, Ex. Adl. DG ICMR, (Chairman).
2. Dr. SK Sharma, Professor and Head, Department of Medicine, AIIMS, (Member).
3. Dr. VK Vijayan, Director Patel Chest Institute, Delhi University Campus, Delhi, (Member).
4. Dr. PP Mandal, CMO Central TB Division, MOHFW, New Delhi, (Member).
5. Dr. PC Bansil, Techno Economic Research Institute, (Member).
6. Dr. ML Srivastava, Techno Economic Research Institute - (Member Secretary).

The first meetings of the Technical Advisory Committee held on 5th June, 2005 at Techno Economic Research Institute, J-7, Saket, New Delhi, discussed, amended and finalized the methodology and study instruments. However, the final shape to study tools was given at a meeting attended by the following and held at CTD, MOHFW on 6–8–05.

Following were present at the meeting held at CTD, MOHFW:

1. Dr. LS Chauhan, Deputy Director General (TB), Central TB Division, MOHFW, Chairman.
2. Dr. Sai Kumar, Consultant WHO.
3. Dr. PP Mandal, CMO Central TB Division, MOHFW, NewDelhi.

3. Dr. Padam Singh, TERI.
4. Dr. ML Srivastava, TERI.
5. Dr. PC Bansil, TERI.

The second meeting of TAC was held on 29th January, 2006 at Techno Economic Research Institute, J-7, Saket, New Delhi. The committee reviewed the progress of the work and finalized the progress report for submission to the sponsors of the study.

7.4.6 Field Work and Data Collection

The field work carried out between July 2005 and August 2006 by specially trained field workers consisting of supervisors and enumerators under the overall supervision of the research team, was organized in a systematic movement format from one DOTS centre/zone to another. This was done to control the quality of data by using a limited field staff over longer period to avoid misinterpretation of instructions. The field team was given intensive training and guidelines, specifically prepared for the purpose for interpretation, understanding and completion of the questionnaires.

7.4.7 Data Processing and Analysis

The completed questionnaires were scrutinized in the office and necessary steps were taken to get reliable and quality information. To facilitate disaggregation and analysis each questionnaire was given one unique six digit identification number. This unique number represented the zone (1st digit), the TB unit (2nd digit), the type of service provider (3rd digit), the type of questionnaire (4th digit) and the selected respondent (5th and 6th digits). Data entry was done using the FoxPro software.

SPSS statistical software package was used for the analysis of data.

7.5 FIELD PROBLEMS

During the course of field work a number of difficulties at the level of service providers and service users were faced. These related mainly to location and cooperation and are given below.

Service Providers

It was difficult to locate a few of the DOTS centers mainly on account of either they were non-functional at the time of the survey or were merged to another one. This shows the need for regular updating of the list of DOTS centers. In all such cases the selected service provider was substituted with another one in the same area to keep the sample size of service providers unchanged. The substitution was effected in six of the ninety cases of service providers in the form of DOTS centers. Of this six, two were found closed, two had insufficient number of cases and were working as sub-centers, one was closed after relocation of the locality and one showed somewhat hostile attitude. The details are given in the footnote of Appendix Table 7.2.

The research/field team faced maximum difficulty in contacting the service providers in "other" category largely in the private sector. The non-cooperation was based mainly on their reluctance to divulge the information about address of patients. Further, most of such service providers in this category were servicing very few patients. This necessitated the reconsideration of the sample of service providers in the "other" category. Taking into account various consideration, it was decided to reconstituted the "other" category to comprise of different types of the service providers including DOTS centers not already considered, both in public and private sectors. The ten service providers included in the sample to achieve the target total sample are listed in Appendix Table 7.3. This difficulty might be kept in consideration while interpreting the results of the study particularly for the service providers in the private sector.

Despite the introductory letter addressed to service providers and issued officially soliciting their cooperation, quite a few were reluctant to allow the field team to carry out work particularly at the exit interview stage. The field staff was, however, able to persuade the DOTS centres belonging to public health sector in all the cases where initial non-cooperation was experienced and the interview proceeded smoothly. The lack of cooperation was more intense at the level of service providers in the private sector than those under the health facilities operated by the official system. The lack of cooperation from the private sector forced the research team to readjust the study-design to include non DOTS service providers in the study.

Service Users

At the time of drawing the sample of service users (cured/completed and defaulted) from the master list maintained at the TU level the addresses were noted down as kept in these records. However, in many cases it was difficult to locate the service users. This was more frequent in the case of defaulters than in the case of cured/completed treatment cases. This might have been largely due to wrong address given at the time of registration, a phenomenon quite common among patients who want to keep their illness secret or who shifted their residence. The shortfall in the sample arising because of this was made up by using a substitute respondent selected initially at the stage of drawing the original sample.

In the case of service users (cured/treatment completed) the cooperation was generally good when located. However, invariably the interview had to be completed quite secretly. This shows the intensity of the taboo that is attached with the disease that people are very much concerned with its nature and would like to keep it hidden. In the case of defaulters, the field staff had to face hostile response in all those cases where some severe side effects were experienced. In other cases the defaulting patients were not that forthcoming in the interaction with the field staff as cured/treatment completed respondents.

SAMPLE PROFILE

7.6 BACKGROUND

The present chapter provides a comparative picture of the socio-economic profiles of TB patients classified in three categories, namely, those who successfully completed treatment, had defaulted or were suspected of the disease. These profiles, where applicable both at patient's and household levels, have also been compared with those for the neighbourhood households without a TB patient but located in the vicinity of patients who successfully completed the treatment and were in our sample.

The presentation first takes up the description of sample relating to each characteristic. At the end, all these data are combined to arrive at a joint score signifying the Socioeconomic Status Index (SES). The discussions of findings and conclusions arrived at later in the subsequent chapters of this book have to be interpreted with this score in perspective. It may be emphasized here that patients who successfully completed treatment or defaulted and were included in our sample were largely drawn from among those who utilized RNTCP services provided mainly by government agencies. These need not necessarily represent the situation in the population at large.

7.7 GENDER AND AGE

Table 7.2 presents the comparison of TB patients in different categories considered here by gender and age. The percentages in the columns relate to respective total sample size in the category. The following observations are worth noting.

- There were relatively more males than females who utilized RNTCP services. This phenomenon was more prominent among the defaulted patients than among those who successfully completed the treatment. The preponderance of males among the defaulted patients could be the reflection of the fact that such patients probably belonged mostly to migrant labour category where they were prone to have come to the city alone. The presence of symptoms of TB among suspected patients by gender conformed more to the

Table 7.2: Respondents by Age, Gender and Patient Category

	Patient Category		
Age (yrs)	*Successfully treated*	*Defaulted*	*Suspected*
0–14	10.6	3.5	10.2
15–24	24.6	24.9	25.3
25–34	36.2	28.1	32.5
0–34	71.4	56.5	68.0
35–44	13.4	21.2	12.1
45–54	8.3	11.1	8.8
>55	6.9	11.2	11.1
>35	28.6	43.5	32.0
Gender			
Male	52.9	70.9	58.5
Female	47.1	29.1	41.5
Total	100.0	100.0	100.0

category of patients who successfully completed treatment than to those who defaulted.

- Male patients in each category considered here used RNTCP services more than female patients. The proportion of males was higher than that of females among those who defaulted (71%) than those who successfully completed treatment (53%). More males than females showed symptoms of TB. The respective percentages were 58.5 and 41.5.
- Treatment compliance by age, like gender, also showed some degree of selective behavior. A clear divide may be noted between those below 35 years and those above this boundary. Among those who successfully completed treatment, about 71% were below 35 years compared to 57% among defaulted patients. Those below 35 years also showed higher chance for contacting the disease as about 68% of those suspected of TB were in this age bracket.
- Defaulted patients were relatively older in age than those in other groups. About 44% of defaulted patients were aged above 35 years compared to 29% of the successfully treated patients in that age bracket.

7.8 CASTE

Table 7.3 presents the distribution of households belonging to different categories of respondents by caste classified into four categories, namely, scheduled castes (SC), scheduled tribes (ST), other backward communities (OBCs), and others. The caste compositions of the neighbourhood households without a TB patient and that of those with a suspected TB patient presented in this table showed the possibility of a higher incidence of the disease among SC/STs. It may be noted that 36% of the households with suspected TB patients belonged to SC/STs compared to 28% of the households without a TB patient. Further, SC/ST appeared more likely to default on treatment compared to patients belonging to OBCs or other castes. It may be seen that 48% of defaulted TB patients belonged to SC/ST category compared to only 32% of those who successfully completed the treatment.

The findings suggest that SCs and STs should be given some special consideration in IEC (Information Education and Communication) activities of RNTCP services. This is expected to improve the treatment compliance in those communities and motivate them for availing treatment.

Table 7.3 shows that RNTCP service users in Delhi come mostly from households belonging to SC/ST/OBC categories. Our sample showed that the share of households belonging to these communities among the total ranged from 66.5% for neighbourhood households to a high of about 83.3% for defaulted patients. Even among the successfully treated patients more than three-quarters of patients (78.2%) belonged to these communities. This share was exceptionally large compared to population of Delhi. This is revealed by data given out by two rounds of NFHS. According to NFHS-3 (2005–06), the caste composition of households in Delhi showed that about one third (32.8%) of the households belonged to these categories. Similar composition was also noted for NFHS-2 (1999) with comparative percentage being 33.5.

Table 7.3: Respondents by Caste and Category

	Category (%)					
	TB Patients			*Neighbourhood Households Without a TB patients*	*Estimate For Delhi**	
Caste	*Successfully completed*	*Defaulted*	*Suspected*		*1999*	*2005–06*
SC	16.3	20.6	16.2	12.8	17.7	17.3
ST	15.7	28.0	20.0	15.4	0.9	1.2
OBC	46.2	34.7	38.8	38.3	14.9	14.3
Others	21.8	16.7	25.0	33.5	66.4	67.2
Total	100.0	100.0	100.0	100.0	100.0	100.0

**Source:* National Family Health Survey-2 Table 2.5 and National Family Health Survey-3, Table 2.3, India, Delhi, IIPS.

7.9 HOUSING CHARACTERISTICS

The information on housing characteristics of households belonging to different categories of respondents is given in

Table 7.4. Frequency of house-ownership was relatively lower among those who were either defaulters or suspected TB patients than among those who either successfully completed treatment or were without a TB patient but were in the neighbourhood. About 58% of households with successfully treated TB patient or without a TB patient but in the neighbourhood were living in accommodations owned by them. By contrast, far fewer about 42–43% of defaulted or suspected TB patients were living in households owned by them. There was a substantially higher percentage among households with defaulted patients than among successfully treated or suspected TB patients who lived in kutcha houses. The respective percentages were 29 against 8 and 10. Further,

Table 7.4: Households by selected characteristics and category of respondents

Selected housing characteristics	*Category (%)*			
	TB Patients			*Neighbourhood households with no TB patient*
	Successfully treated	*Defaulted*	*Suspected*	
Ownership				
Owned	57.4	41.5	43.3	58.0
Rented	42.6	58.5	56.7	42.0
Type of house				
Pucca	91.2	70.8	89.6	92.8
Katcha	8.8	29.2	10.4	7.2
Number of rooms				
1	56.6	66.4	65.6	57.2
2	39.3	29.4	24.8	34.2
>2	4.1	4.2	9.6	8.6
Independent room for patient				
Available	6.6	6.3	5.5	Not applicable
Not available	93.4	93.7	94.5	Not applicable
Total	100.0	100.0	100.0	100.0

households with defaulted TB patients and suspected TB patients had fewer rooms as compared to those who successfully completed treatment and those living in neighbourhood households. For example, 66 to 69 percent of households with defaulted or suspected TB patients lived in housing units with 1 room as against 55% and 57% for other two categories. The degree of crowding appeared to be quite high in each category as more than half of the households managed their affairs in one room dwelling units. As a result only about 6–7% of the households could afford independent room for the TB patients. Such a high incidence of crowding is likely to expose more people to the risk of catching the infection of TB.

7.10 SOURCE AND TREATMENT OF DRINKING WATER

The distribution of households by source of drinking water and its treatment before use presented in Table 7.5 showed close similarity for each of the four categories of respondents. About 80 to 85 percent of the households were drinking water supplied by the Delhi Jal Board. Since this water is already treated, it does not necessarily require any further treatment. However, the remainder of the households depended upon

Table 7.5: Households by source of drinking water, method of treating It and category of respondents

Water, source and treatment characteristics	*Category (%)*			
	TB Patients			*Neighbourhood households with no TB patient*
	Successfully treated	*Defaulted*	*Suspected*	
Source of water				
Well	0.8	0.5	0.7	1.1
DJB	85.7	82.5	84.4	82.7
Hand pump	13.5	17.0	14.9	16.1
Water treatment				
Boil water	2.0	0.7	1.2	2.2
Aquaguard	0.2	2.3	0.7	1.4
None	97.8	97.0	98.1	96.3
Total	100.0	100.0	100.0	100.0

water for drinking drawn from hand pumps and needed some treatment in order to protect the users from water born diseases. The data did not show any action on this account as almost the entire population living in these households used water as was available from the source.

7.11 TOILET FACILITY

Table 7.6 presents information on the availability of toilet facility to households belonging to different categories of respondents. Relatively higher percentage of households with defaulted patients or suspected TB patients compared to those in other two categories were sharing toilets or defecating in the open. Separate toilets were available to about 28% and 24% of households with defaulted and suspected TB patients. By contrast, about 40% of households with successfully treated patients had separate toilet facility. The comparative figure for neighbourhood households was only 31%.

Table 7.6: Households by toilet facility and category of respondents

	Category (%)			
	TB Patients			*Neighbourhood households with no TB patient*
Toilet facility	*Successfully treated*	*Defaulted*	*Suspected*	
Separate	39.0	27.7	23.8	31.1
Shared	52.9	62.7	69.6	60.1
Public	6.5	7.0	3.8	7.6
Open place	1.4	2.6	3.1	1.2
Total	100.0	100.0	100.0	100.0

7.12 FUEL USED FOR COOKING

Table 7.7 presents data on fuel used for cooking in households covered by the survey. It may be mentioned that higher percentage of households with defaulted patients (30%) and suspected T.B patients (24%) were using kerosene oil for cooking as compared to other two categories (about 18 to 19 percent). The most popular fuel used for cooking is identified as liquefied petroleum gas (LPG). Almost two-thirds to four-fifths of the households were dependent on LPG for cooking purposes.

Table 7.7: Households by type of fuel used for cooking and category of respondents

Fuel for cooking	*Category (%)*			
	TB Patients			*Neighbourhood households with no TB patient*
	Successfully treated	*Defaulted*	*Suspected*	
Firewood	0.9	1.9	1.7	1.1
Kerosene	19.3	30.1	23.5	18.4
Gas	78.4	66.7	73.8	79.8
Others	1.4	1.4	1.0	0.7
Total	100.0	100.0	100.0	100.0

7.13 WORKING STATUS

A comparison of the results on the working status of patients and monthly income of households with such patients in three categories is presented in Table 7.8. Of the three categories of TB patients considered here, relatively higher proportion among defaulted TB patients were daily wage earners. About

Table 7.8: Respondents by work status and category and their households by monthly income

Working status	*TB Patient*		
	Successfully treated	*Defaulted*	*Suspected*
Daily Wage worker	14.8	26.1	18.2
Monthly wage worker	22.1	19.9	24.3
Not working	63.1	54.0	57.5
Monthly household income (Rs.)			
<2000	14.4	19.6	18.1
2000-3000	35.3	51.2	37.9
3000-4000	40.6	23.0	37.9
>4000	9.7	6.2	6.1
Total	100.0	100.0	100.0

26% of the defaulted patients were daily wage earners as compared to 15% and 18% of the successfully treated and suspected patients. Those in the non-working group (students and housewives) were more among those who successfully completed treatment. About 63% of the successfully treated patients were not working as compared to 54% of defaulted patients and 58% of suspected patients. Also, those in the category of defaulted TB patients had lower income as compared to TB patients who successfully completed treatment. Only about 29% of the households with defaulted patients had income exceeding Rs 3,000 per month. By contrast, about 50% of households with successfully treated patients and 44% of households with suspected TB patients belonged to this group.

7.14 HOUSEHOLD ASSETS

The distribution of assets owned by neighbourhood households in comparison with those with TB patients in the three categories is presented in Table 7.9. Following observations are worth mentioning.

- Among the various assets identified, the top spot was taken by fan. This was followed by radio and TV, respectively, at the second and the third place. Fourth place was taken by fridge whereas the cycle occupied the fifth place.

Table 7.9: Households by type of assets possessed and category of respondents*

	Category (%)			
	TB Patients			*Neighbourhood households with no TB patient*
Type of assets possessed	*Successfully treated*	*Defaulted*	*Suspected*	
Fan	89.9	87.5	86.1	86.2
Radio	58.3	56.9	58.0	62.0
Fridge	22.0	11.3	18.6	24.7
TV	59.8	44.4	48.8	64.2
Phone	1.5	0.5	0.9	4.4
Cycle	16.9	12.0	12.5	14.0
Vehicle	5.0	3.0	1.5	6.6
Grinder/mixer	4.0	1.9	2.8	5.9

*Multiple response.

- Possession of fan or radio showed little variation among the households in different categories. The percentage of households with fan to total in various categories considered varied between 86 to 90 percent whereas that for the radio varied between 57 and 62. The variation in percentage of households with TV was large. The households with defaulted and suspected patients were similar with 44% and 49% households having a TV. Similar pattern may be noted for the other two categories with respective percentages as 60 and 64 for households with successfully treated patients and in the neighbourhood.
- The ownership of high value assets (TV, fridge) was more in neighbourhood households not having any TB patients than in households belonging to other three categories. About 25 and 64 percent of households in the neighbourhood of successfully treated patients possessed fridge and TV respectively. The next category was households with successfully treated patients with comparative percentage as 22 and 60 respectively. The lowest figures were for the households with defaulted patients where 11 and 44 percent of households possessed these assets.
- The four wheeler vehicle and grinder/mixer were also reported more among neighbourhood households compared to other three categories.
- The households with TB patients who successfully completed treatment were relatively closer to the neighbourhood households without a TB patient in respect of possession of high value assets.
- The number of households with defaulted TB patients or that with those suspected of TB and not availing treatment was relatively fewer in possessing such assets.

7.15 SOCIOECONOMIC STATUS (SES) INDEX

Based on the information in respect of sample households regarding type of house, type of occupancy, main source of lighting, source of drinking water, type of fuel used, toilets and household possessions presented earlier in this chapter, a composite Socioeconomic Status (SES) Index was computed. This index gives an idea of the relative level of quality of life that different groups of respondents enjoyed. This index, suggested by TNHSP, uses a set of weights. Table 7.10 presents the various details about the definition and the computation of the index.

The score is designed to range between 0, signifying the lowest level of living to 54, the highest level of living, all consistent with the scope of information used in its computation. To facilitate interpretation and collective assessing these have been classified in to five nominal categories, namely, lowest, low, medium, high and highest, as specified at the bottom of Table 7.10.

It might be noted from the combined SES score given in Table 7.10 that there was a close similarity in the households that were in the sample. However, scores showed a negligible but rising trend in SES index for households with defaulted, suspected and successfully treated TB patients in that order where the total score increased from 21.8 for households with defaulted patients to 23.8 for those with successfully treated patients. Households with suspected patients occupied a place in between the two with a score of 22.6. It may be noted, however, that households belonging to each group of patients fall in low SES category. By contrast, neighbourhood households without a TB patient belonged to medium SES category, though the score was only marginally higher than that for those households which had successfully treated patients. One tentative conclusion which is likely here is that TB patients who benefit from RNTCP programme are generally from low socio-economic category. Further, those who are likely to benefit more from the program are somewhat better of socially and economically than those who default or neglect themselves.

Table 7.10: Computation of socio-economic status index

		Successfully treated		*Defaulted*		*Suspected*		*Neighbourhood households with no TB patient*	
Category/Items	**Weight**	**%**	**Score**	**%**	**Score**	**%**	**Score**	**%**	**Score**
Type of House									
Kutcha	0		0		0		0		0
Semi-pucca	2	8.2	16.4	29.2	58.4	10.4	20.8	7.2	14.4
Pucca	4	91.2	364.8	70.8	283.2	89.6	358.4	92.8	371.2
Type of Occupancy									
Own house	4	57.4	229.6	41.5	166	43.3	173.2	58	232
Rented house	2	42.6	85.2	58.5	117	56.7	113.4	42	84
Temporary shelter	0		0		0		0		0
Main Source of Lighting									
Electricity	2	100	200	100	200	100	200	100	200
Kerosene/oils	1		0		0		0		0
Source of Drinking Water									
Piped water, well water, ground water (in home)	2	85.7	171.4	82.5	165	84.4	168.8	82.7	165.4
piped water, well water, ground water (public)	1	0.8	0.8	0.5	0.5	0.7	0.7	1.1	1.1

Contd...

Table 7.10: Computation of socio-economic status index (*Contd...*)

		Successfully treated		*Defaulted*		*Suspected*		*Neighbourhood households with no TB patient*	
Category/Items	**Weight**	**%**	**Score**	**%**	**Score**	**%**	**Score**	**%**	**Score**
Surface water	0	13.5	0	17	0	14.9	0	16.1	0
Type of Fuel Used									
LPG/biogas	2	78.4	156.8	66.7	133.4	73.8	147.6	79.8	159.6
Coal/Coke/lignite/ kerosene	1	19.3	19.3	30.1	30.1	23.5	23.5	18.4	18.4
Wood/Crop residues/ Dung Cakes	0	0.9	0	1.9	0	1.7	0	1.1	0
Toilets									
inside house	3	39	117	27.7	83.1	23.8	71.4	31.1	93.3
outhouse	2	52.9	105.8	62.7	125.4	69.6	139.2	60.1	120.2
public	1	6.5	6.5	7	7	3.8	3.8	7.6	7.6
no facility	0	1.4	0	2.6	0	3.1	0	1.2	0
Household Possessions									
Pressure Cooker	1	100	100	100	100	100	100	100	100
Mixer/Grinder	3	4	12	1.9	5.7	2.8	8.4	5.9	17.7
Steel Cupboard	1	100	100	100	100	100	100	100	100

Contd...

Table 7.10: Computation of socio-economic status index (*Contd...*)

		Successfully treated		*Defaulted*		*Suspected*		*Neighbourhood households with no TB patient*	
Category/Items	**Weight**	**%**	**Score**	**%**	**Score**	**%**	**Score**	**%**	**Score**
Water pump	2	0	0	0	0	0	0	0	0
Cot or bed/Mattress	1	100	100	100	100	100	100	100	100
Fan	2	89.9	179.8	87.5	175	86.1	172.2	86.2	172.4
TV	2	59.8	119.6	44.4	88.8	48.8	97.6	64.2	128.4
Radio/Transistor	2	58.3	116.6	56.9	113.8	58	116	62	124
Sewing machine	2	30	60	30	60	30	60	30	60
Telephone	3	1.5	4.5	0.5	1.5	0.9	2.7	4.4	13.2
Refrigerator	3	22	66	11.3	33.9	18.6	55.8	24.7	74.1
Bicycle	2	16.9	33.8	12	24	12.5	25	14	28
Moped/Scooter/Motorcycle	3	5	15	3	9	1.5	4.5	6.6	19.8
Car	4	0	0	0	0	0	0	0	0
Bullock Cart	2	0	0	0	0	0	0	0	0
Tractor	4	0	0	0	0	0	0	0	0
Total score per unit			23.8		21.8		22.6		24.0

Contd...

Table 7.10: Computation of socio-economic status index (*Contd...*)

		Successfully treated		*Defaulted*		*Suspected*		*Neighbourhood households with no TB patient*	
Category/Items	**Weight**	**%**	**Score**	**%**	**Score**	**%**	**Score**	**%**	**Score**
Socioeconomic Status Category			Low		Low		Low		Medium
Basis of Categorization	SES Category								
Score 1–12	Lowest								
score 12–24	Low								
score 24–36	Medium								
score 36–48	High								
> score 48	Highest								

Appendix Table 7.1: Distribution of DOTS cum microscopic centres and DOTS centers by zone and TB unit along with sample allocation of DOTS centers

Zone	*TB unit*	*DOTS Cum Microscopic*	*DOTS Centre*	*DOTS Centre*	
				Total	*Sample*
West	RK Mission	6	5	11	3
	Moti Nagar	5	12	17	4
	DDU Hari Nagar	10	13	23	6
	RTRM Jaffar Pur	9	11	20	5
	Sub Total	**30**	**41**	**71**	**18**
North	Gulabi Bagh	10	11	21	3
	Kingsway Camp	7	8	15	3
	BJRM Jahangir Puri	6	5	11	3
	SGM Mangolpuri	13	10	23	4
	Narel Lampur Road	5	19	24	5
	Sub Total	**41**	**53**	**94**	**18**
East	Patparganj	7	11	18	4
	Shahdara	5	15	20	4
	GTB Shahdara	6	8	14	3
	Karawal Nagar	6	7	13	3
	Hedgewar Karkardooma	5	12	17	4
	Sub Total	**29**	**53**	**82**	**18**
South	LRS Mehrauli	15	13	28	9
	Nehru Nagar	15	16	31	9
	Sub Total	**30**	**29**	**59**	**18**
Central	Jhandewalan	4	3	7	3
	NDMC	5	4	9	3
	NDTB	2	2	4	3
	Lok Nayak Hospital	4	0	4	2
	Sub Total	**15**	**9**	**24**	**11**
Old Delhi	SPM Marg	6	18	24	7
	Sub Total	6	18	24	7
All Zones	Total	151	203	354	90
	Other Service Providers	–	–	–	10
Delhi	Total Sample	–	–	–	100

Appendix Table 7.2: List of DOTS centers selected in the sample by zone and TB unit, Delhi 2005

	TB unit	Seliected DOTS Centers
West Delhi		
1.	Chest Clinic RK Mission DOT Cum Microscopy Centres	1. RK Mission, 2. Budh Nagar and 3. Baljeet Nagar
2.	Moti Nagar DOT Cum Microscopy Centres	1. Moti Nagar, 2. Lakkar Mandi and 3. Arora Moti Nagar, 4. F-Block Madipur
3.	Deen Dayal Uppadaya Hospital DOT Cum Microscopy Centres	1. DDU Hari Nagar, 2. Palam Village (Colony), 3. Pratap Garden, 4. Janak Puri, 5. Sagarpur and 6. Mayapuri, Ind. Area-II.
4.	RTRM Hospital, Jaffar Pur DOT Cum Microscopy Centres	1. RTRM Jaffarpur, 2. A-Block Kakrola, 3. Vikas Nagar, 4. Prem Nagar B-Block, and 5. Shyam Vihar
North Delhi		
5.	Gulabi Bagh DOT Cum Microscopy Centre	1. Gulabi Bagh, 2. Ashok Vihar Phase-I, and 3. MCD Sara Basti
6.	Kingsway Camp DOT Cum Microscopy Centre	1. RBTB Kingway Camp, 2. Sangam Park, and 3. Shankracharya Marg,
7.	BJRM Hospital, Jahangirpuri DOT Cum Microscopy Centre	1. BJRM Jahangir puri, 2. Jahangirpuri, B-Block and 3. Basti Vikas Kender
8.	SGM Hospital, Mangolpuri DOT Cum Microscopy Centre	1. SGM, Mangol Puri, 2. Jawala Puri, 3. Sultanpuri and 4. A.mangolpuri.
9.	Narela DOT Cum Microscopy Centre	1. Narela Lampur Road, 2. Barwala Delhi, 3. Shahabad Dairy, 4. Daryapur Kalan, and 5. Bhorgarh Village
East Delhi		
10.	Patparganj DOT Cum Microscopy Centre	1. Patparganj, 2. Trilok Puri, 3. Lal Bahdur S. Hospital1, 4. Mandavali
11.	Shahdara DOT Cum Microscopy Centre	1. Chhota Bazar Shahdra, 2. Raghuver Pura - I, 3. Raghuverpura-I, and 4. Krishna Nagar
12.	GTB Hospital Shahdara DOT Cum Microscopy Centre	1. G.T.B Shahdra, 2. Seema Puri and 3. Sundar Nagari
13.	Karawal Nagar DOT Cum Microscope Centre	1. Karawal Nagar, 2. Arvind Nagar and 3. East Gokul Puri
14.	Hedgewar Chest Clinic DOT Cum Microscope Centre	1. Hedgewear, 2. Karkardoma, Geeta Colony, 3. Laxmi Nagar and 4. Maharam Mohalla
South Delhi		
15.	LRS Institute	1. LRS Mehrauli, 2. Delhi Khanpur,

Contd...

Appendix Table 7.2: List of DOTS centers selected in the sample by zone and TB unit, Delhi 2005 (*Contd...*)

	TB unit	*Seliected DOTS Centers*
	DOT Cum Microscopy Centre	3. Sangam Vihar, J- Block, 4. Fateh Pur Beri, 5. Jaunapur Village, 6. Rajokri, 7. Vasant Kunj, 8. Madangir (I-Block) and 9. Sangam Vihar (J Block)
16.	Nehru Nagar DOT Cum Microscopy Centre	1. Nehru Nagar, 2. Sarai Kale Khan, 3. Madan Pur Khadar, 4. Garhi, 5. Batla House, 6. CASP, 7. World vision, 7. Govind Puri and 9. Harkesh Nagar
Central Delhi		
17.	Chest Clinic Jhandewalan DOT cum Microscopy Centre	1. Jhande Walan, 2. Sadar Bazar and 3. Kishan Ganj, Chamelian Road.
18.	NDMC DOTCum Microscopy Centre	1. Shaheed Bhagat Singh Marg, 2. Aurangzeb Lane and 3. Lajpat Nagar
19.	NDTB DOT Cum Microscopy Centres	1. HDTB, Jawaharlal Nehru Marg, 2. Sita Ram Bazar and 3. Vakil pura
20.	Chest Clinic Lok Nayak Hospital DOT Cum Microscopy Centre	1. Jawahar Lal Nehru Marg, 2. Jama Masjid
Old Delhi		
21.	Chest Clinic SPM Marg DOT Cum Microscopy Centre	1. SPM Marg, Pili Kothi 2. Sabsi Mandi, (Hindu Rao Hospital) 3. Laori Gate, Lalkuan, 4. Malka Ganj 5. Kashmiri Gate, 6. Shah Ganj and 7. Gali Samosa (Fresh Khana)

Appendix Table 7.3: List of additional service providers to make the complete total sample size

DOTS Centers

1. Jain Charitable Hospital, Raghuvera Pura – II Gali No. 5.
2. Private Service, Jain Charitable Hospital Raghuvera Pura – II, Gali. No. 5, Charge per day per patient Rs.10.
3. Delhi Government DOTS Centre Chhattarpur.
4. Delhi Government DOTS Centre Ber Sarai
5. Delhi Government DOTS Centre Malviya Nagar
6. Wasu Memorial Charitable Dispensary, Sainik Farms, charge per patient per day – Rs.10/-
7. DOTS Center, AIIMS
8. DOTS Center, Kingsway Camp Hospital
9. DOTS Center LRS Mehrauli
10. Patel Chest Institute, Delhi University Charge per day per patient Rs. 10–15/-

8

Treatment Seeking Behaviour

8.1 INTRODUCTION

Successful completion of, default or negligence in seeking treatment for any patient is largely dependent on her/his contextual behavior, perception of the problems associated with the disease in question, cost of and convenience with which the services are available. The understanding of this aspect in a community receives more relevance in our case as treatment of TB is generally sought without disclosing the identity of the patient. This attitude generally follows from social and other stigma attached to the disease. For successful implementation and efficient operation of RNTCP it was considered useful to understand the behavior of the TB patients toward the above factors. Therefore, in our survey an attempt was made to seek information on a few factors which could help us to assess the status of patients in respect of factors that were responsible for their behaviour and understand the dynamics of undertaking treatment to total, partial or no action at all. The factors can be linked to what motivates the patients to take particular action on the one hand and on what emotional and functional difficulties are faced in using these services on the other. Our investigation covered the following factors:

- Source of advice for seeking treatment.
- Treatment availed earlier.
- Delay in initiating treatment.
- Choice of DOTS center for treatment.

- Distance of DOTS center.
- Mode of transport to DOTS center.
- Person normally accompanying the patient to DOTS center.
- Time use pattern in the context of getting service at DOTS center.
- Current health status of patients.

The findings are presented respectively in sections 8.2 through 8.12 of this chapter.

8.2 SOURCE OF ADVICE FOR SEEKING TREATMENT

The question, "who motivated the patient to seek medical help", was included in the questionnaire to understand the role of motivators in persuading patients to accept the treatment for TB. The findings are presented in Table 8.1 which covers two categories of patients, that is, those who successfully completed the course and those who defaulted on the treatment each split in three groups-adult male, adult female and child.

Family members appeared to play the most important role in convincing patients to seek TB treatment. In about 72–85 percent of the cases, depending upon the category of patients, family members were helpful in convincing the patients to seek treatment. This is quite expected in the case of children where in 85% of the cases family members advised in favour of treatment for successfully treated patients. In the case of defaulted child patients the family members appeared to play somewhat less important role with about 73% being in this group. The health personnel played a far distant second placed role in 9 to 13 percent of the cases in convincing the patient/family for seeking medical help. In about 10% of the cases involving successfully treated children, health personnel played a role in helping the family to seek medical help. The comparative percentage for defaulted child-patients was 13.

Like the case of child patients, family again played the most dominant role in seeking medical help in the case of adult patients. The decision to seek medical help in the case of adult male and adult female patients, irrespective of the fact whether they completed successfully or defaulted, was based on the advice of family members. About three-quarters of the patients sought medical help on the advice of family members. However, the role of family was marginally more important in the decision in respect of adult female patients than male patients. Similar pattern was observed in respect of the role of health personnel who occupied a distant second place in advising patients to seek medical help. This was noted in about one of ten cases. Further, adult males and females showed some degree of independence and took decision to seek medical help on their own. However, as expected adult males showed somewhat greater flexibility in taking decision compared to adult female patients. For example, about 8% of adult male patients took the decision to seek medical help on their own compared to only 6% of the successfully treated adult female patients. The differential in the case of defaulted patients was only one percentage point.

With one exception, neighbours, co-workers or community leaders apparently played negligible role in the decision of patients to seek medical help. In the case of defaulted adult male and female patients neighbours appeared to play some role in convincing them to seek medical help. This possibly could be the reflection of the social stigma attached to the disease as patients and families tried to keep the incidence of disease as secret. The details are given in Table 8.1.

Table 8.1: Successfully treated and defaulted TB patients (adult male, adult female and child) by source of advice for seeking TB treatment*

Source of advice for seeking treatment	*Category of patients (%)*					
	Successfully treated			*Defaulted*		
	Adult			*Adult*		
	Male	*Female*	*Child*	*Male*	*Female*	*Child*
Own/Self	8.1	5.8	Na**	8.2	7.2	Na**
Family member	76.9	78.2	85.3	71.5	76.8	73.4
Neighbours	3.6	3.2	2.0	6.2	8.0	6.7
Co-workers	1.7	1.0	Na**	1.6	0.8	Na**
Health personnel	9.2	11.2	9.5	8.9	8.8	13.3
Community leaders	0.0	0.4	0.4	0.3	0.0	0.0

* Multiple responses

** Na = not applicable

- In view of the dominant role played by family members in convincing patients to seek TB treatment, it is advisable to target the family members in the IEC activities of the RNTCP more intensively.
- Efforts should be made toward increasing the role of community in motivating people in general to be conscious of the disease and to seek medical help available free of cost through DOTS centers.

8.3 TREATMENT AVAILED EARLIER

The programme for arresting the spread and curing the already infected patients of TB through DOTS strategy under RNTCP could be implemented more effectively and efficiently if we had the information on what patients did about the disease prior to coming to the DOTS center. To assess this aspect a question on the prevalence of such practice was included in our survey. Also, in such cases where any prior medical help was taken, the source of such treatment was ascertained. The findings are presented in Table 8.2 for the comparable categories as in Table 8.1.

Here it may be noted that nearly 18% of the patients (17.7% of the successfully treated and 17.6% of the defaulted ones) had availed treatment from other hospitals/dispensaries, private practitioners before coming to DOTS centers from where they were sampled. Of these, about 77% of total patients, successfully treated as well as defaulted, availed earlier treatment from Government hospitals and dispensaries, 8% from private practitioners, 6% from Rotary/NGO run clinics and remaining ones from other service facilities (Table 8.2). Table 8.2 shows broadly a similar pattern for successfully treated adult males, adult females and children with about four-fifths of them getting treated at government hospitals/ dispensaries prior to coming to the present DOTS center.

Relatively higher share of children and adult females than adult males among defaulted TB patients availed treatment from Government Hospitals and Dispensaries before coming to the current DOTS centers. Among the defaulted patients, about 10% of adult males as opposed to no child-patients

Table 8.2: Successfully treated TB patients (adult male, adult female, child and total) by source of treatment if availed earlier

Source of treatment if availed earlier	Category of patients (%)							
	Successfully treated				Defaulted			
	Adult				Adult			
	Male	Female	Child	Total	Male	Female	Child	Total
Government hospital/ dispensary	76.8	77.5	84.2	77.0	75.8	80.8	86.7	76.8
Private practitioner	8.6	7.9	3.6	8.3	9.5	4.0	0	7.9
Rotary/NGO	6.9	6.1	7.2	6.3	5.3	7.2	6.7	6.0
Private hospital	1.0	1.0	1.6	1.0	0.3	0.8	0	0.6
Others	6.7	7.5	3.4	7.4	9.1	7.2	6.6	8.7
Total	100.0	100.0	100.0	100.0	100.0	100.0	100.0	100.0

and 4% of adult females received treatment from private practitioners. The data show the tendency for preference, though not substantial, in favour of males in getting treatment from private practitioners before coming to the DOTS center. It is more a reflection of the fact that adult males who are generally the bread winner for the family receive somewhat higher preference in attending to their health problems. About one in every ten adult male patient compared to far fewer adult female and child patients get treatment from private practitioners before attending the DOTS center.

8.4 DELAY IN INITIATING TREATMENT

Delay in seeking treatment is likely to be harmful to the patient as well as to the community. This attitude can have quite serious implications particularly in the case of tuberculosis which is infectious and debilitating, among other complications, in nature. To know what factors affect people's behaviour in delaying such a step, the survey collected data on the factors that cause delay in seeking help to treat TB using DOTS facilities that are provided free of cost by the government to any patient. We consider the three groups of patients (successfully treated, defaulted and suspected) in the following three sub-sections to present our findings. The nine reasons covering social, psychological, economic and infrastructural issues for successfully treated and defaulted patients and five for suspected patients were considered for data collection. Of these, only two, namely, "initial concealment of the disease" and "not aware of DOTS centers providing cost-free treatment" were most important. The remaining seven were cited by negligible percentage of patients. The findings are summarized in Tables 8.3 to 8.5.

8.4.1 Successfully Treated TB Patients

Of the successfully treated TB patients, about one-sixth reported some delay in initiating treatment from DOTS center. Table 8.3 clearly shows the dominant role of only two of the nine reasons that account for delay in seeking treatment. The dominant reasons for this delay were mainly "the initial concealment of the disease" (72.5%) and "lack of awareness of the DOTS centers providing free treatment" (65%).

Such a high incidence of initial concealment possibly results from the stigma attached to the disease. Somewhat similar, though slightly, lower incidence of lack of awareness about DOTS centers providing free treatment is somewhat surprising in communities where about 60% of households possessed a TV or a radio set. This finding suggests that vital public health programme such as TB control is not receiving enough publicity in electronic media. This suggests that there is a need to use these mass media sources more productively to increase people's awareness in specified areas of concern.

The distribution of patients who successfully completed treatment by reasons for delay in getting treatment, separately for adult males, females and children is given in Table 8.3.

The initial concealment of disease as a reason for delay in seeking treatment was reported higher among adult female patients and children as compared to adult male patients, the respective percentages were 73.7, 76.8 and 68.0. However, "not aware of DOTS Centers providing free treatment" was reported as the main reason for delay by almost the same percentage of adult male, adult female patients (65%). In the case of child patients this reason was reported by a slightly higher percentage at about 69.

Table 8.3: Successfully treated TB patients (adult male, adult female, child and total) by reasons for delay in initiating treatment*

	Category of patients (%)			
Reasons of delay in initiating treatment	*Male*	*Female*	*Child*	*Total*
Initial concealment of the disease	68.0	73.7	76.8	72.5
Indecision on where to take treatment	1.0	0.3	0.4	0.6
Negligence of family members	0.7	0.4	0.4	0.5
Financial problem	0.2	0.3	0.4	0.4
Pressure of work	0.6	0.3	0.4	0.4
Symptoms not severe enough	0.6	0.2	0.4	0.3
Distance of the service provider	0.3	0.3	0.4	0.3
Not aware of DOTS center providing free treatment	64.9	65.0	68.7	64.7
Non availability of service provider	0.3	0.3	0	0.3

*Multiple response

8.4.2 Defaulted TB Patients

Like successfully treated patients, of those who defaulted on the treatment for TB, about one sixth reported some delays in initiating treatment from DOTS center they were captured in the sample. The reasons behind this action were, again like the successfully treated patients, mainly "initial concealment of the disease" (75%) and "not aware of the DOTS centers providing free treatment" (62%). The incidence of other reasons for delay to get the treatment initiated was negligible at less than one percent (Table 8.4).

As pointed out earlier, since a large percentage of households of defaulted patients possessed TV and/or Radio, it would be useful to intensify the current IEC programme accordingly to convey the information that free treatment for TB was available through DOTS centers.

Results on delay in getting treatment for defaulted TB patients, separately for adult males, females and children given in Table 8.4 showed that the initial concealment of disease as a reason was reported higher among adult female patients (77%) and children (80%) as compared to adult male patients (71%). "Not aware of DOTS Centers providing free treatment" was reported as the main reason for delay by about 62% of adult males and females and about 67% of children.

Table 8.4: Defaulted TB patients (adult male, adult female, child and total) by reasons for delay in initiating treatment*

	Category of patients (%)			
Reasons of delay in initiating treatment	*Male*	*Female*	*Child*	*Total*
Initial concealment of the disease	70.8	76.8	80.0	75.2
Indecision on where to take treatment	0.3	1.6	0	0.7
Negligence of family members	0.3	0.8	0	0.5
Financial problem	1.0	0.8	0	0.9
Pressure of work	1.0	0.8	0	0.9
Symptoms not severe enough	0.7	0.8	0	0.7
Distance of the service provider	0.5	0.8	0	0.7
Not aware of DOTS center providing free treatment	61.6	62.4	66.7	61.6
Non availability of service provider	0.0	0.0	0.0	0.7

*Multiple response

8.4.3 Suspected TB Patients

The main reason reported for not availing treatment was that they were either not aware of free treatment available from DOTS center (more than 80%), or not sure of the disease as TB (more than 25%). Negligence of family members was more prominent in the case of children (23%) than that in the case of adult males (14%) and adult females (12%). Pressure of work and loss of wages, as expected, primarily came in the way of males seeking treatment for the disease. Too costly to afford private treatment was also a prominent reason for not availing treatment particularly in the cases of adult males and adult females (Table 8.5). The diversity of reasons for neglecting the treatment in the case of suspected patients compared to those who received either full or partial treatment at DOTS centers points to lack of awareness about the services provided by government totally free of cost for the treatment of TB. This finding again suggests the need for strengthening the awareness raising programmes.

Table 8.5: Suspected TB patients (adult male, adult female and child) by reason for not seeking treatment*

Reasons for not getting treatment	Precent		
	Adult Male	Adult Female	Child
Not sure of disease as TB	25.0	26.3	25.6
Not aware of free treatment at DOTS centre	81.0	80.7	86.0
Too costly to afford private treatment	8.1	7.0	2.3
Negligence of family members	13.7	12.3	23.3
Pressure of work and loss of wages	10.9	4.1	4.7

*Multiple response

8.5 CHOICE OF DOTS CENTER FOR TREATMENT

The choice of DOTS center by patients for treatment of TB is likely to be affected by a number of factors. We identified ten of them. These were: good care, proximity, availability of expertise, equipment, cost free quality drugs, confidentiality, convenient working hours, etc. One factor which was considered initially but subsequently deleted from the list related to relatives/acquaintances working in the place because it got a negligible about 3% response only in the case of defaulted female patients. This response was only 3.2 percent. Other ten reasons for the selection of particular DOTS center or the service provider are given in Table 8.6 for the various categories of patients considered here. While interpreting data it may be taken into account that multiplicity of reasons for the selection of DOTS center was possible.

Cost-free service was the dominant reason for selection of DOTS center for treatment. This was reported by about three-quarters of the successfully treated and six-tenths of the defaulted TB patients. Convenient working hours, proximity and good care were other three reasons which could influence patient's choice to substantial extent. It was interesting to note that convenience of working hours though an important factor in the choice of DOTS center was also the most important factor

Table 8.6: Successfully treated and defaulted TB patients (adult male, adult female, child and total) by reasons for selecting the DOTS center/service provider where treatment was undertaken*

Reasons for selecting the DOTS center	Category of patients (%)							
	Successfully treated				Defaulted			
	Adult Male	Adult Female	Child	Total	Adult Male	Adult Female	Child	Total
Good care /attention	29.3	29.9	22.6	27.4	17.0	18.4	26.7	17.4
Proximity	23.2	25.4	19.0	24.1	16.4	19.2	26.7	17.1
Availability of expertise	2.8	2.8	3.2	2.8	1.6	3.2	6.7	2.1
Availability of equipment	1.9	2.0	2.8	2.0	1.3	3.2	6.7	1.9
Convenient working hours	65.0	65.7	71.0	65.3	27.9	24.8	33.3	25.0
Quality of drugs	2.9	2.7	3.2	2.8	3.3	3.2	6.7	3.2
Minimum waiting time	4.4	4.2	5.2	4.3	3.9	6.4	6.7	4.6
Cost free	75.5	76.2	70.6	75.7	59.0	63.2	66.7	60.0
Confidentiality	4.4	5.1	4.4	4.7	3.0	4.0	6.7	3.2
Neighbours	1.7	1.6	2.0	1.7	0.3	3.2	0	1.2

*Multiple Response

in differentiating the successfully treated patients from those defaulted on the treatment. Where about 65% of the successfully treated patients perceived that working hours were convenient, only 25% of the defaulted patients found the working hours convenient. This observation assumes significance in the sense that to promote completion of the treatment course it might be necessary to look in to the convenience of patients in respect of the working hours. Good care and proximity were the reasons for the selection of the particular DOTS center for about one-quarter of the successfully treated patients. By comparison only about 17 percent of the defaulted patients found these factors favourable for selection of particular DOTS center. DOTS centers under government set-up generally opened at

8.30 in the morning and closed at 2.30 in the afternoon. Most of the poor patients who had to go for work early in the morning and return home late in the evening found it difficult to avail the services, although free. To improve the utilization of DOTS centers it might be useful to widen the working hours, at least for distribution of medicines, which were more convenient to working patients. In this context it may be noted that some of the DOTS centers which had a NGO social worker were able to provide services to these labourers according to their convenience.

The distribution of successfully treated patients by reasons for selecting DOTS Centre for treatment was very much similar for adult males and adult females. In the case of children, however, there was some variation. Working hours, however, were found more convenient in the case of successfully treated children (77%) than that in the case of adult males (65%) and adult females (66%). The difference in percentage points in favour of children was about 5 points. Good care/attention, proximity and cost free treatment as reasons for selection of DOTS center were reported by fewer successfully treated children (71%) than adult males and adult females (76%) in that category.

The comparative picture of reasons for selection of DOTS center for adult males, adult females and children in the defaulted category was somewhat different from that of successfully treated patients. Relatively higher proportion in case of children compared to adult males and females reported cost free treatment, good care/attention, proximity, and convenient working hours as reasons for selecting DOTS centers for treatment. For example, about 67% of children as opposed to about 59% adult males and 63% adult females among defaulted patients cited "cost free" as a reason for the selection of DOTS centers for treatment of TB. This was at variance with successfully treated patients where children generally accounted for lower percentages than adult males and adult females among such patients cited varying reasons for the selection of DOTS centers. The exception is only the cost free provision.

8.6 DISTANCE OF DOTS CENTER

RNTCP has a policy to provide TB treatment facilities within easy reach of the beneficiaries. This is possible only when the establishments are easily accessible or are located within walking distance with reference to the residence of patients. In this context a distance of one or two km from the residence could be considered short enough for easy access. To assess this factor we collected data on the distance which the patients had to cover to reach the DOTS center. The results of the analysis are presented in Table 8.7. In this case we have considered the total number of patients without any consideration of the gender or age. However, we have differentiated the successfully treated patients from those who defaulted on the treatment.

It may be noted in Table 8.7 that DOTS centers were generally within easy reach of the patients. Of the successfully treated patients about 62% had to cover a distance of 1 km and additional 30% had to travel a distance of up to 2kms. A very low percentage of such patients (8%) had to cover more than 2 km to reach the DOTS center.

Table 8.7: Distance of DOTS centre from residence of successfully treated and defaulted TB patients

Distance of DOTS Centre (Kilometer)	*Category of patient (%)*	
	Successfully treated	*Defaulted*
1	61.6	56.6
2	30.0	34.0
>2	8.4	9.4
Total	100.0	100.0

Defaulted patients, on the average, appear to cover marginally greater distance but more than 90% were located within 2 km of the DOTS centers. This comprised of 57% and 34% of the defaulted patients who were living within 1 and 2 km of the DOTS centers.

8.7 MODE OF TRANSPORT

The earlier information on the distance of the DOTS centers from the residence of each patient supplemented with that on the mode of transportation used to reach there provides a comprehensive picture of the access of such centers to patients. We present in Table 8.8 the data on the mode of transport used by patients of different categories.

As demonstrated in Table 8.8 more than 80% of the patients, either successfully treated or defaulted, walked to the DOTS center and/or took a rickshaw or other such similar facility to reach there. About 45% of the successfully treated patients and 50% of the defaulted patients walked to the centers whereas respectively 36% and 32% of these patients used a rickshaw or similar such facility. Travel by bus to the DOTS center occupied a distant third rank with 12% of the successfully treated patients using this means of transport. Fourth place was taken by bicycles accounting for about 6% of the successfully treated patients. These two modes of transport interchanged their ranks in the case of defaulted patients with 8% and 7% going to the DOTS centers by cycle and bus respectively.

Table 8.8: Mode of transport normally used by successfully treated and defaulted TB patients (adult male, adult female, child and total) while going to the service provider/DOTS center

Mode of transport used	*Category of patients (%)*							
	Successfully treated				*Defaulted*			
	Adult Male	*Adult Female*	*Child*	*Total*	*Adult Male*	*Adult Female*	*Child*	*Total*
On foot	43.9	46.5	46.4	44.5	49.2	52.0	53.3	50.1
Cycle	7.8	0.0	4.4	5.7	9.8	0.0	0.0	8.1
Scooter	2.4	4.7	1.6	1.9	2.3	1.6	0.0	2.1
Auto	0.6	0.4	0.4	0.5	0.3	0.8	0.0	0.5
Bus	12.2	10.9	9.9	11.5	6.2	8.0	13.3	6.9
Rickshaw and Others	33.1	37.5	37.3	35.9	32.2	37.6	33.4	32.3
Total	100.0	100.0	100.0	100.0	100.0	100.0	100.0	100.0

When the mode of transport used for reaching the DOTS centers is analyzed for adult males, adult females and children some expected patterns emerge. The pattern of the mode of transport used by adult males is somewhat different from that for adult females and children. For example, use of bicycle was largely confined to adult males where it accounted for attendance to DOTS center of about 8% of the successfully treated patients and 10% for defaulted patients. The use of this means in the case of children is largely the reflection of the fact that they were accompanied by adult males who escorted them to the center.

One observation which needs to be made here is, though the DOTS centers were located within 2 km of the residences of over 80% of the patients, about one-half or slightly more reported the use of some means of transport to reach the center. This implies some expenditure which had to be met from their already low incomes as would be seen later on in this book.

8.8 PERSON NORMALLY ACCOMPANYING THE PATIENT TO THE SERVICE PROVIDER

Table 8.9 presents the distribution of successfully treated and defaulted patients in each category by type of relationship to the patient of the person who normally accompanied the patient to the service provider. This is essential to understand the social behaviour in Indian society where it is assumed that, at least in the case of adult females and children, some one will escort the patients to the medical center.

In majority of the cases, as is clear from Table 8.9, patients went to the service provider unaccompanied. This may be noted in the case of 54% of the successfully treated patients and 61% of the defaulted ones. This large share of patients going to the DOTS center unaccompanied was dominated by the case of adult males in both the categories of patients as more than 71% of the males went to the center unaccompanied. By comparison only 29% and 32%, respectively, of successfully treated adult female patients and defaulted adult female patients were unaccompanied. The incidence of small percentage of children going to the center unaccompanied may be explained on the ground of the proximity of the centers to the residences. If the

Table 8.9: Successfully treated and defaulted TB patients (adult male, adult female, child and total) by type of relationship to person normally accompanying the patient to DOTS center/service provider

Type of relationship to patient	Category of patients (%)							
	Successfully treated				Defaulted			
	Adult Male	Adult Female	Child	Total	Adult Male	Adult Female	Child	Total
Spouse	5.2	23.7	Na	13.8	7.5	31.2	Na	14.4
Son	2.9	8.9	Na	5.7	6.6	14.4	Na	8.8
Daughter	0.2	0.6	Na	0.1	0.0	0.0	Na	0.0
Father	1.5	2.0	6.0	1.7	2.0	2.4	20.0	2.1
Mother	17.8	35.8	83.7	24.4	9.2	18.4	73.3	11.8
Brother	1.0	0.4	0	0.7	1.3	1.6	0.0	1.4
Sister	0.2	0.0	1.2	0.1	0.0	0.0	0.0	0.0
Friend	0.1	0.0	Na	0	0.3	0.0	Na	0.2
Nobody	71.1	28.6	9.1	53.5	73.1	32.0	6.7	61.3
Total	100.0	100.0	100.0	100.0	100.0	100.0	100.0	100.0

Na = Not applicable

centers were located very close to the residences, it was quite possible that children, particularly those close to the end of the age group, could be sent alone to receive medication.

Mother, spouse or son were three important categories of close relationships in that order of importance who accompanied the patients. The respective shares were 24%, 14% and 6% in the case of successfully treated patients. The comparative percentages for defaulted patients were 12, 14 and 9.

Gender and age showed some strong differentials in the pattern of escorts to the DOTS centers. As noted earlier males were largely unaccompanied. By contrast, as expected, adult females and children were largely accompanied by some one. In the case of children, mother normally accompanied the patient. This may be noted in the case of 84% of the successfully treated children as compared to only 6% of them who were accompanied by the father. The comparative figures for defaulted patients were 73 and 20. Thus more than 90% of the children were accompanied by either the mother or the father.

In the case of adult females, as expected, only about 29% of the successfully treated ones and 32% of the defaulted ones went to the DOTS centers unaccompanied. About 69% of the successfully treated adult female patients were accompanied by either the mother (36%), spouse (24%), or son (9%). The pattern of relationship of the escort to the patient for the defaulted adult female patients was somewhat at variance with that for the successfully treated adult female patients. Whereas in the case of successfully treated adult female patients, mothers played the dominant role as escort the same was not true for defaulted patients. Here spouse played the dominant role with escorting about 31% of the defaulted adult female patients. Additional 14% were escorted by their sons. Mothers escorted only 18% of the patients in this category. The point worth noting that emerged here related to the role of the relationship of the escorts to the patients in the successful completion of treatment. In the absence of mother escorts in substantial cases for defaulted adult female patients, accompanying husbands and sons needed some counseling in the importance of sustained attendance at the DOTS centers and completion of the course of treatment. This is expected to encourage them to escort the female patients to the service providers.

It may be noted that in the case of 93% of defaulted children mother or father, as expected, normally accompanied the patient to the service provider whereas in the case of about two-thirds of adult females, spouse, mother or son generally accompanied the patient. Counseling of parents is expected to promote the treatment compliance in the case of child-patients. About 73% of defaulted adult males and 32% of defaulted adult females went to the service provider unaccompanied. The intensive counseling programmes for patients as well as for escorts are to be encouraged for improved compliance of treatment.

8.9 TIME USE PATTERN IN THE CONTEXT OF GETTING REGULAR SERVICE

As pointed out earlier our sample largely came from the lower socio-economic groups and therefore the requirement on the time of patients to get medicines and attend the DOTS center on a regular basis played an important role in their compliance. In this background we assessed the perception of TB patients about the time use pattern in getting the services at such centers. The information on the length of time required to attend regularly the DOTS center and the perception of reasonableness of this time are respectively presented in Tables 8.10a and 8.10b.

Table 8.10a: Successfully treated and defaulted TB patients by time required for attending the DOTS centre

	Category of patient (%)	
Time required (hours)	*Successfully treated*	*Defaulted*
1	79.7	79.9
2	15.4	3.5
>2	4.9	16.6
Total	100.0	100.0

Table 8.10b: Successfully treated and defaulted TB patients by perception about length of waiting time in getting treatment and convenience of working hours at the DOTS centre

		Category of patient (%)	
Characteristic	*Perception*	*Successfully treated*	*Defaulted*
Waiting time	Long	5.3	6.3
	Reasonable	94.7	93.7
Working hours	Convenient	93.7	9.0
	Inconvenient	6.3	91.0
	Total	100.0	100.0

About 80% of the patients in each of the two categories took up to one hour in going to the DOTS center and receiving medicines. The remaining ones showed somewhat different patterns for the time that they needed to complete the routine. Whereas only about 5% of the successfully treated patients needed more than 2 hours to travel and get their regular supply of medicines, about 17% of the defaulted ones fell in this category.

Most of the patients found the waiting time reasonable. The percentages of successfully treated and defaulted patients which fell in this group were 95 and 94. However, when we examine the pattern of perception of working hours we notice a radical difference between the two groups of patients. Whereas only about 6% of the successfully treated patients found the time inconvenient, more than 90% of the defaulted patients found the timings of the centers inconvenient. This observation implies that inconvenience of time of the clinics could be a contributing factor for default. In this context it may be noted that all the DOTS centers worked from 8.30 AM to 2.30 PM. This timing could be quite inconvenient for poor people who had to go for work early in the morning and return late in the evening. To increase compliance this problem was tackled through programmes in selected centers where morning and evening services were provided by NGOs. This participation between the government services and the NGOs, has improved the compliance rate in centers benefiting from this. It is important to consider extension of working hour, at least for distribution of regular medicines. This is expected to improve the compliance rate.

8.10 CURRENT HEALTH STATUS

The collective information on "feeling of wellness" after successful treatment or default can be fed-back in the system to promote/encourage patients for completion of the entire course or convince them to continue in treatment if already entered. It is in this context that the study enquired about the current health status of both the categories of patients. The resulting data are presented in Table 8.11 and observations are summarized below.

About 95% of successfully treated patients felt that they were completely cured. A similar percentage of such patients had presumably recovered fully and resumed their normal work. By contrast, of the defaulted patients only 51% felt that they were completely cured. The percentage of such patients who felt that they had recovered fully and resumed normal work was somewhat higher than percentage of those who felt they were completely cured. The respective percentages were 67, 70 and 51. This discrepancy between feeling cured on the one hand and feeling fully recovered and resumption of normal duties might be explained on the basis of economic pressure as most of the male patients were expected to be working. But in the sense of its implication, this discrepancy is serious as these patients might still be active careers of the disease. Their mixing with healthy people may have serious health implications and needs to be handled carefully through counseling.

Feeling of completely cured or fully recovered does not appear to be universal even after successful completion of the treatment course. Of all the successfully treated patients about 6% reported that they were still having some health problems and 11% experienced a decline in their efficiency. The corresponding percentages for the defaulted patients were understandably much higher than this. Of all such patients about 36% still had some health problems at the time of survey and 27% were experiencing decline in their efficiency.

Results on "Current Health Status" for successfully treated patients presented in Table 8.11 revealed a somewhat similar pattern for each of the three categories considered here (adult male, adult female and child) as for the total. This conclusion

Table 8.11: Successfully treated and defaulted TB patients (adult male, adult female, child and total) by current health status*

	Category of patients (%)							
	Successfully treated				*Defaulted*			
Current health status	*Adult Male*	*Adult Female*	*Child*	*Total*	*Adult Male*	*Adult Female*	*Child*	*Total*
Completely cured	94.8	95.0	98.4	94.9	50.5	52.0	33.3	50.7
Some health problem persists	5.3	5.9	3.2	5.6	28.2	24.8	66.7	35.9
Recovered fully	94.8	94.5	96.4	94.3	66.6	70.4	66.7	67.4
Resumed normal work	95.2	95.4	97.8	95.4	69.8	70.4	33.3	69.7
Decline in efficiency	10.7	12.4	9.5	11.4	27.2	22.4	25.0	27.1

* Multiple response

however is not true for defaulted patients. Relatively lower proportion among children compared to adult males and adult females reported as completely cured and consequently higher proportion of them reported having continued health problems. Only one-third among children reported resuming normal work as against 70 percent among adult males and females.

8.11 REASONS FOR DEFAULT

To improve the compliance rate among TB patients who are under treatment it might be useful to asses the reasons for default as well as the health status after they discontinue the medication. These aspects will help in understanding the dynamics of default and make suitable modifications in our approach to patients. The survey made an attempt in this direction and the results relating to the reasons for default are summarized in this section whereas those relating to the health status after default and at the time of survey are presented in the following section.

Table 8.12 presents the distribution of defaulted TB patients by reasons for default. With reference to the total patients it

Table 8.12: Defaulted TB patients (adult male, adult female, child and total) by reasons for default*

	Adult			
Reasons for default	*Male*	*Female*	*Child*	*Total*
No effect of treatment	27.2	32.0	33.3	28.5
Feeling cured	48.5	39.2	46.7	45.6
Too costly to afford	0.3	2.4	0.0	0.9
Finding it difficult to go to service provider	4.9	6.4	6.7	5.3
Time schedule for collecting medicines not convenient	46.3	42.9	43.2	44.6
Pressure of work and loss of wages	6.9	2.4	0.0	5.6
Nobody to escort	1.6	1.6	0.0	1.6
Symptoms subsides	2.3	4.0	0.0	2.8

*Multiple response

may be noted that main reasons for default were "feeling cured" (46%), "time schedule for collecting medicines not convenient" (45%) and "no effect of treatment" (29%). Pressure of work and loss of wages as reason was reported by only 6% of the defaulted patients. Reasons related to service providers, i.e. "finding difficult to go to service provider" reported by 5% of the defaulted patients together with about 45% who found "time schedule for collecting medicines inconvenient" stood at about 50%. A negligible 3% of the respondents reported that they discontinued the treatment because symptoms of the disease subsided.

The pattern of reasons for default given by adult males, females and children showed some variation, though the three main reasons for default remained the same. In the case of "no effect of treatment" as a reason for default, it was lowest for the adult males (27%) and highest for children (33%). In the case of the other two main reasons adult females occupied the intermediate position between adult males on the higher side and the children on the lower side. Where about 49% of adult males and 47% of children reported that they defaulted because they were feeling cured, about 39% of adult females did that. The comparative percentages for the "time schedule for collection of medicines inconvenient" were 46, 43 and 43 respectively. "Pressure of work and loss of wages", as a reason for default, as expected, was reported mainly by adult males (7%). Reasons related to service providers in respect of their location was reported more in the case of adult females and children than in the case of adult males. The reasons related to service providers combining the two (location and timing) for defaulting on treatment in the case of adult males at 51% was somewhat similar to that for adult females (49%) and children (50%).

The analysis of reasons for default has brought three main reasons for an action. These are: "feeling cured", "time schedule for collection of medicine not convenient" and "no effect of treatment". These can broadly be grouped in to two, one relating to the operation of services and another relating to misunderstandings. It may be recalled that 91% of defaulted patients had earlier reported that timings of the DOTS centers were "not convenient" to them. This observation together with the fact that about 45% of such patients dropped out of system because of the inconvenience of the time schedule for collection of medicines should be given serious thought by the RNTCP services. There is a strong need for providing medicines at hours convenient to most of the patients as they are from lower working classes.

Another action which the Programme should consider is about the counseling of patients. It appears that after initial treatment they feel to have become well and drop from the system. It is appropriate that each patient is accordingly counseled and properly followed-up to ensure continued participation in the system. "No effect of treatment" as a reason for default appears to be serious and needs careful follow-up. The medical reasons for "no response of the medication" at individual level must be ascertained and remedial action taken. This will boost the confidence level of patients in the system.

8.12 STATUS AFTER DEFAULT

To improve the treatment compliance it is useful to assess the status of defaulted patients after they left the system. The survey attempted to find out the extent of any attempt made by the programme to track such patients as well as to get an idea of their health and work status and whether the patients knew the implications of their action. The resulting data are summarized in Table 8.13.

It is encouraging to note that the RNTCP system had a policy of follow-up in case of default. However, the intensity of this action does not seem to match the requirement. Only 26% of the defaulted patients admitted that they were contacted to continue the treatment. There was hardly any difference between the experiences of follow-up contact among different groups of patients as the percentages of contacted patients varied between 25 for adult females to 27 for children. It appears there are logistical difficulties in following-up all the defaulted cases because of wrong addresses and relocation of patients but this makes a strong case for counseling at the time patients are brought in to the system.

Table 8.13: Status of defaulted TB patients (adult male, adult female, child and total) after defaulting on treatment*

Status after default on treatment	*Adult*			
	Male	*Female*	*Child*	*Total*
Contacted for continuous treatment	26.9	24.8	26.7	26.2
Current feelings				
Very well	20.0	18.4	20.0	19.4
Well	52.5	47.2	40.0	50.7
Not well	27.6	33.6	40.0	29.9
Able to work normal hours	33.1	26.4	20.0	31.0
Knows that the incomplete treatment can harm	23.0	16.8	20.0	21.1
Willingness to complete treatment	11.8	6.4	13.3	10.2

*Multiple responses.

The perception of health status was assessed by their feelings at the time of survey. It may be noted that about 30% of total defaulted patients reported "not well", 51% as "just well" and only 19% reported as "very well". From the programme's perspective the intensity of "not well" needs special consideration on two counts. One, it should serve the purpose for convincing the in-coming patients that incomplete treatment could harm their health in the long run. Two, it should impress on the authorities to take remedial action so that these people did not become agents for negative publicity of the Programme. The perception of "not well" was more among children (40%) than among adult males (28%) and adult females (34%). This finding may indicate that children and females are not given that much care as males.

After giving up treatment, about 31% of the total defaulted patients were able to work normal hours. Relatively more adult males (33%) than adult females (26%) and children (20%) were able to work normal hours. This finding is reflecting the pattern of feeling "not well" in the sense that those who felt well were able to work normal hours than if they felt "not well".

Over 20% of total defaulted patients knew that incomplete treatment could prove harmful. This awareness was relatively better among adult males (23%) and children (20%) as compared to adult females (17%). About 10% were willing to complete their treatment but did not get family support. Willingness to continue treatment was also higher among adult males (12%) and children (13%) as compared to adult females (6%).

9

Economic Implications

9.1 COVERAGE OF ECONOMIC IMPLICATIONS

Tuberculosis because of its infective nature has many costs to the individual as well as to the family and community. Since the disease is associated with several stigmas generally linked with its debilitating effects, it has heavy economic burden as well. The worst affected is the family. Additional burden falls on the community and the government because it causes a lot of disruptions in economic activity of the individual. In the context of our study we have examined the impact of the disease on the following:

- Employment
- Working hours
- Job change
- Income
- Duration of treatment
- Expenditure related to disease
- Financing of treatment
- Financial burden of illness

9.2 EMPLOYMENT

The responses received from successfully treated and defaulted patients on their employment status before, during and after treatment are summarized in Table 9.1. This is expected to reflect on the possible impact of the disease on this important aspect of family finances as quite a high proportion of patients were bread-winners for the family. The impact is measured by the deviation of proportion in gainful employment before illness with that during and after illness. The deviation is expected to provide the magnitude of the impact of the disease on the employment status. It may be noted that, before illness, among those who successfully completed treatment, about 64% constituted the group of students, housewives and unemployed; the remaining about 36% of employed comprised of 14% on "daily wage employment", 19% "in service" and 4% "self-employed". The percentage of employed during treatment phase declined by about 12 percentage points mainly amongst wage earners and those in service. Thus, only about 70% of the successfully treated and employed patients continued in the job during the treatment phase. Consequently, the percentage of housewives, students and unemployed among such patients during the treatment phase increased to about 76. It is heartening to note, however, that after the treatment the employed status reverted to almost the original status.

Table 9.1: Successfully treated and defaulted TB patients by employment status before, during and after treatment

	Category of patients and stage of treatment (%)					
	Successfully treated			*Defaulted*		
	Stage of treatment			*Stage of treatment*		
Employment status	*Before*	*During*	*After*	*Before*	*During*	*After*
Wage employment	13.5	10.2	12.5	26.3	23.5	23.5
Service	18.8	11.7	18.8	18.8	17.0	16.5
Self employed	3.7	2.3	3.9	4.0	3.3	3.3
Housewives, students unemployed	64.0	75.8	64.8	50.9	56.2	56.7
Total	100.0	100.0	100.0	100.0	100.0	100.0

The picture among the defaulted patients is somewhat different. In this group there were more employed persons before the start of the treatment than among the successfully treated ones. It may be obtained from Table 9.1 that, compared to about 36% employed before start of treatment among successfully treated patients, the relevant percentage among the defaulted patients was about 49. Among those who defaulted on treatment, only about 51% were students, housewives and unemployed; 26% were on daily wage employment, 19% were in service and 4% were self employed. The employment status distribution clearly brings out the most important structural difference in this characteristic for the two group of patients. The daily wage employment is the main differentiating factor between the two groups. It seems those on wage employment if caught by the disease are quite likely to default. One possible reason for default in this group could be based on their temporary stay in the city where they come for wage employment and after falling prey to the disease either go back or relocate themselves about which we have no clue. This inference is consistent with the fact that the percentage of defaulted patients living in rented accommodations at about 59% was 16 points higher than that for those who were successfully treated (Table 7.4). The percentage of unemployed among such patients increased during as well as after incomplete treatment by over five points mainly from amongst wage earners and those in service. The continued high percentage of wage employment among defaulted patients during as well as after incomplete treatment appears to be reflection of some genuine difficulty for such patients to stay under treatment. One factor which could be worth investigation is that such patients found it difficult to continue despite the fact that they were aware of the dangers of their action.

9.3 WORKING HOURS

The successfully treated patients, who were wage earners or in service, generally worked for eight hours (about 80%). In one fifth of these cases, the working hours were longer than eight hours. Strong structural adjustment in working hours during the treatment phase for successfully treated patients is indicated for those who continued in employment. This is indicated by the substantial increase in percentages of those working eight hours (about 90% of employed) and drop in percentage for those working more than eight hours. However, it was encouraging to note some degree of recovery to original status of length of working hours after the treatment. About 85% of the employed patients worked for eight hours per day.

Like successfully treated patients, defaulted ones also generally worked for eight hours (about 80% of the employed defaulted patients). In one fifth of such cases the working hours were longer than eight hours. There was a sharp drop among those working for more than eight hours during disease phase, which continued even after treatment. This shows that defaulted patients failed to regain their strength to revert to normal working hours (Table 9.2).

Table 9.2: Successfully treated and defaulted TB patients by length of working hours per day before, during and after treatment

Length of working hours per day	*Category of patients and stage of treatment (%)*					
	Successfully treated			*Defaulted*		
	Stage of treatment			*Stage of treatment*		
	Before	*During*	*After*	*Before*	*During*	*After*
Not applicable	64.0	75.8	64.8	50.9	56.3	56.7
8 Hours	28.6	21.8	30.1	41.0	39.0	40.0
>8 hours	7.4	2.4	5.1	8.1	4.7	3.3
Total	100.0	100.0	100.0	100.0	100.0	100.0

9.4 JOB CHANGE

Besides length of working hours per day, the change in job is another factor which the disease is likely to affect. However, tuberculosis appeared to play practically negligible role in this respect during the illness phase. Change in jobs among the successfully treated patients during treatment phase was reported by only some 2.0% where about 24% of the total were engaged in some kind of wage/salary employment. Despite the increase in percentage employed among such patients after treatment (35% as opposed to 24% during treatment phase) very few (less than one percent) reported change in job at this stage (Table 9.3).

Incidence of change in job among the defaulted patients was even less than that among successfully treated ones. As is clear from Table 9.3 only 2% of the defaulted patients where 44% were employed experienced a change in job during the treatment phase. This figure declined further to almost negligible level after they defaulted on treatment. The lack of any major shift in job structure during or after treatment is probably the reflection of the rigid occupational opportunities in the area of study.

Table 9.3: Successfully treated and defaulted TB patients by whether any change in their Job during and after treatment

Whether change in job	*Category of patients and stage of treatment (%)*			
	Successfully treated		*Defaulted*	
	Stage of treatment		*Stage of treatment*	
	During	*After*	*During*	*After*
Yes	2.1	0.7	1.9	0.6
No	22.1	34.5	42.6	42.8
Not applicable/no response	75.8	64.8	55.5	56.6
Total	100.0	100.0	100.0	100.0

9.5 INCOME

The average monthly income of the employed and successfully treated patients was Rs. 2,730 per person before illness. It was reduced to Rs. 2,650 during treatment phase but went up to Rs. 2,790 after treatment (Table 9.4). Thus, for the successfully treated patients the average income per month per working patient shows some variation from one to other phase of treatment. The dip in income during the treatment phase is worth noting. By contrast, the effect of disease in terms of income per month per patient shows marked impact. In the case of successfully treated patients the average income per month per patient during the treatment phase declined from a level of Rs. 980 in pre-treatment phase to Rs. 640 during treatment phase, a dip of Rs. 340 per month per patient. It reverted to Rs. 980 per month per patient after the treatment phase, this was almost the same as before the treatment phase.

Defaulted patients showed somewhat different averages. Income per month per employed defaulted patient declined to Rs. 2390 during the treatment phase from Rs. 2620 during

Table 9.4: Successfully treated and defaulted TB patients by monthly income in rupees by stage of treatment–before, during and after

Monthly income in rupees	*Category of patients and stage of treatment (%)*					
	Successfully treated			*Defaulted*		
	Stage of treatment			*Stage of treatment*		
	Before	*During*	*After*	*Before*	*During*	*After*
Not applicable	64.0	75.8	64.8	50.9	56.3	56.7
<1000	1.0	0.8	0.3	2.6	3.6	1.2
1000-2000	8.7	7.1	8.6	7.2	12.8	15.2
2000-3000	12.0	6.8	11.7	24.4	15.4	14.0
3000-4000	10.2	7.3	10.2	12.4	9.6	11.1
4000-5000	3.5	1.6	3.7	1.6	1.4	1.4
>5000	0.6	0.6	0.7	0.9	0.9	0.4
Total	100.0	100.0	100.0	100.0	100.0	100.0
Average income						
Per employed	2731	2649	2788	2620	2388	2438
Per patient	983	641	982	1287	1044	1056

*Not applicable

pre-treatment phase, a dip of Rs. 230 per month. Unlike successfully treated patients, the average monthly income of employed and defaulted patients after the default on treatment remained almost similar to that during treatment phase at about Rs. 2440. Since the defaulted category of patients had larger proportion of them employed or working, the average monthly income per defaulted patient before treatment at Rs. 1280 was higher than that for successfully treated patients by about Rs. 300 per month. The unfavourable difference increased to about Rs. 400 per month during the treatment phase and declined drastically to Rs. 80 during the phase after default. It may be mentioned that the income per month per defaulted patient registered a fall to the level Rs. 1040 during the treatment phase and small increase to Rs. 1060 after the default on treatment. This shows that whereas successfully treated patients registered the recovery to the level of income as before treatment the defaulted patients did not show that characteristics.

9.6 DURATION OF TREATMENT

The duration of treatment for successfully treated patients, as expected under the regime of treatment recommended, was largely six months. This was noted for 87% of such patients and 8 months for 12% of the cases. Only a few had to continue treatment beyond 8 months (Table 9.5).

Table 9.5: Successfully treated TB patients by duration of treatment

Duration of treatment in months	*Percent*
6	86.9
8	11.9
>8	1.2

The duration for which the defaulted patients took treatment is expected to reveal the pattern of continuing with the course of medication. The distribution of length of treatment as given in Table 9.6 shows a wide variation. The default began as early as one month when about one-quarter of the patients stopped taking medicines. By the end of two months cumulatively almost 60% of them had stopped taking medicines. And by the end of three months about eight in ten defaulted patients had stopped medication.

Table 9.6: Defaulted TB patients by duration of treatment (months)

Duration of treatment (months)	*Percent*
1	25.0
2	33.6
3	20.8
4	9.3
5	5.6
>6	5.7

Two aspects of this distribution need to be examined. One, those who stopped taking medicines by the end of three months and two, those who went beyond this but did not complete the course even when they continued as long as 6 months. The first group consists of those who apparently feel better and thus consider themselves cured and did not think further medication was needed. This group has to be guided for continuation. It is necessary that this information should be incorporated in the counseling and patients should be informed. This is the dangerous category because they ignore the significance of going through the complete course. A determined effort needs to be made to track these patients and ascertain causes for default and take necessary steps to overcome them. Needless to add that the benefits of this tracking would go a long way for the success of RNTCP.

9.7 EXPENDITURE RELATED TO DISEASE

Despite the fact that entire medication and related diagnostic expenses are cost-free to the patients under the DOTS system, it was noted that patients had to bear some incidental expenses. The survey attempted to determine the type and extent of such expenses. It may be noted in Table 9.7 that as high as 93% of the successfully treated patients reported incurring expenditure on additional food and the average monthly expenditure under this head was about Rs. 300 (Table 9.8). Further, about 19% of such patients reported expenditure on travel, the average being about Rs. 88 per month. Those reporting expenditure on drugs, pathological labs and consultations were less than 5%. There were a few private DOTS Centers like Jain Charitable Trust

Table 9.7: Successfully treated and defaulted TB patients incurring expenditure by item*

	Category of patients (%)	
Item of expenditure	*Successfully treated*	*Defaulted*
Travel	18.8	15.7
Drugs	4.5	3.5
Pathological Tests	3.0	1.2
Consultant	0.8	0.5
Additional Food	92.7	73.1
Escort Travel	0.7	2.1

*Multiple response

that charged Rs. 10 per day from their private patients who did not like to go to the free DOTS Centre located on the first floor in the same premises, but preferred paying a nominal fee possibly due to stigma attached to the disease.

The pattern of items of expenditure for defaulted patients was somewhat different from that for successfully treated ones. In this case as high as 73% of defaulted patients reported incurring expenditure on additional food (Table 9.7) and the average expenditure per month under this head was about Rs. 225 (Table 9.8). Further about 16% reported monthly expenditure on travel, the average being about Rs. 80. Those reporting expenditure on drugs, pathological tests and consultations were less than four percent.

Table 9.8: Successfully treated and defaulted TB patients by monthly expenditure on additional food for patient

Monthly expenditure on additional food in Rupees	*Category of patients (%)*	
	Successfully treated	*Defaulted*
Nil	7.3	0.3
0–50	0.4	1.3
50–100	7.8	23.0
100–150	2.9	1.0
150–200	24.3	29.7
200–300	20.6	18.4
300–400	13.0	9.3
400–500	9.9	8.9
500–1000	11.4	8.1
>1000	2.4	0.0
Total	100.0	100.0
Average (Rs.)	298	225

9.8 FINANCING OF TREATMENT

Since the successfully treated as well as the defaulted patients had to incur expenditure during the treatment period on items other than medicines, it was relevant to determine the source of such financing. The average extra expenditure on such items, while under treatment for the entire duration of treatment per successfully treated patient, was assessed at about rupees 2,130. The information on mode of financing these extra expenses is summarized in Table 9.9. It may be noted that in 92% of the cases, it was met from the savings in the household. In some cases (2%) loan had to be taken. Assistance was also received from friends and employers in a few cases.

For defaulted patients the average extra expenditure on items other than medication during the period under treatment was obtained at about rupees 1130. Table 9.9 shows that in 72% cases, it was met from the savings in the household. In some cases loan had to be taken. Assistance was also received from friends in few cases. The difference between the percentages of successfully treated and defaulted patients on account of previous savings being used for meeting extra expenses during the course of treatment implies the shaky financial background of the defaulted patients. It raises the question whether the financial instability leads to default on treatment.

Table 9.9: Successfully treated TB patients by source of financing the treatment

	Category of patients (%)	
Source of financing	*Successfully treated*	*Defaulted*
Previous saving	92.2	71.8
Loan	1.8	1.4
Pledging/Sale of assets	0	0.0
Friends	1.1	0.2
Employer	0.2	0.0
Medical Insurance	0.0	0.0
NA/NR*	4.7	26.6
Total	100.0	100.0

*Not available / no response

9.9 FINANCIAL BURDEN OF ILLNESS

We noted earlier that of the total patients who successfully completed treatment, only about 36 percent had wage employment before and after illness. During illness 12 percent of such patients went out of wage employment. The average monthly income before illness of these patients was Rs. 2,730 per worker which got reduced to Rs. 2,640 during illness. After illness the income reverted to almost the same level as before. This implies that during illness period, in addition to complete income loss of 12 percent of TB patients, there was a reduction amounting to Rs. 80 (Rs. 2730 – Rs. 2650) per worker per month in the earning capacity of patients who remained in the wage employment (Table 9.4). Using this data, total loss of wages for 12 percent working patients thrown out of job during illness period and reduced incomes for the remaining 24 percent of them, it is calculated that the average wage loss per month per wage earning patient because of illness was about Rs. 960 (Rs. 958) per month.

To assess the impact of tuberculosis on financial requirements, it would be useful to convert the above loss in to some kind of neutral figure. This can be done by relating the loss to all the patients irrespective of wage employment status. This we can do by calculating the monthly income in respect of each successfully treated patient. As shown in Table 9.4 we may note that the income per month per patient before illness was Rs. 983 which got reduced to Rs. 641 during illness. Thus, the difference amounting to Rs. 342 may be assigned to the loss due to illness in earning capacity per patient irrespective of employment status.

Further, during illness period, about 93% of successfully treated patient, on an average, spent about Rs. 298 per month per patient (Table 9.8) on additional food and nutritious diet. Additionally, nineteen percent of successfully treated patients spent about Rs. 88 per month per patient on travel etc (section 9.7). These expenses may be normalized as before for comparative purpose and the expenditure per patient irrespective of whether expenditure made or not, may be obtained as Rs. 277 and Rs. 17 on additional food and transport etc per month. Thus, the financial burden on the patients' household may be calculated as Rs . 636 (Rs. 342 + 277 + 17) per month. On the assumption of seven months average for the course of treatment, the financial burden of Rs. 4,450 per successfully treated patient during the treatment period is arrived at,. Of this burden, 54% was due to wage loss, 43% could be accounted by additional food and remaining 3% by expenditure on travel, etc. (Table 9.10).

Table 9.10: Successfully treated TB patients by pattern of financial burden on the household*

Type of burden	*Rs.**	*Percent*
Wage less	2394	54
Additional Food	1939	43
Travel	119	3
Total	4452	100

*Rupees per household for an average duration of treatment of seven months.

It may be noted that the above estimate does not take in to account expenses on pathological tests, etc. medical assistance received from outside the DOTS system and the cost of such items when in the system. Thus the actual cost of treating one tuberculosis patient to successful completion and complete recovery may be much more than what we have given above. The other factors have to be accounted for when calculating the cost of the disease per patient at the national level. This must take into account direct expenses incurred by patients, the costs met out of the government medical system of DOTS and the costs under the DOTS system.

10

Socio-Psychological Aspects

10.1 INTRODUCTION

Tuberculosis, because of stigma attached to the disease, usually inflicts quite heavy toll on social life and psychological conditions of the patient. The patient experiences some sort of mental torture and social isolation. In this context it is useful to understand the extent of such experiences and, if possible, to design and implement counter measures to facilitate the participation of patients and communities in the control and eventual eradication of the disease. The survey, therefore, attempted to collect data from patients in three categories (successfully treated, defaulted and suspected) on varied subjects ranging from discrimination at various levels to treatment of family and others toward the patient to the impact of the disease on the education and rearing of children. The findings are presented in Sections 10.2 through 10.4. The successfully treated and defaulted patients, because of several commonality and comparability, are considered in one section whereas the suspected ones are placed separately. The scope of questioning for the two groups also had some distinct differences. Where possible the factors are analyzed for adult males, adult females and children along with the total. Such an analysis helped us to identify the differences in patient's and people's perceptions about the disease and the personal sentiments.

To assess the impact of the disease without confounding it with other factors the experiences and feelings were found with reference to three time-period, namely, before the onset of the disease, during the period of the disease and after either successful completion or the default as the case was faced in particular situations.

10.2 SOCIAL COSTS

To understand the social costs that patients had to bear the survey concentrated on ten factors. These are:

Discrimination within community/caste

- General
- Social function/marriage
- Stigma about marriages

Discrimination within family

- Discrimination in food
- Separate room for living
- No mixing with children
- Discord in marital status
- Isolated in family

Others

- Sunned by co-workers
- Mental depression of the patient

The resulting data for successfully treated and defaulted patients, total as well as three groups mentioned, are given in Table 10.1.

10.2.1 Successfully Treated and Defaulted Patients

It is clear from Table 10.1 that incidence of tuberculosis has a distinct social and psychological toll on the patient during the disease phase. In the case of successfully treated patients we note almost negligible socio-psychological pressure on the patient either before or after the disease phase. The exception with negligible importance is the marital discord and mixing with children, both understandable. It might be observed that during disease phase about one in every 5 TB patients, who successfully completed treatment, faced stigma in terms of discrimination in food, the discomfort of not mixing with children, discord in marital relationship and mental depression. During the same phase close to one in every ten patients felt left out by community in general in the place they lived as well as in social functions/marriages. A similar percentage faced community/caste stigma about marriages even at the family level. The low incidence of discrimination in residence accounted for only about one in twenty patients is understandable, though desirable, in the light of non availability of separate room for patients. The incidence of "isolation in the family" and "shunned by co-workers" was negligible. It is satisfying to note, however, that after the treatment, patients did not face any of these problems and reverted back almost to the same status as before on-set of the disease.

The incidence of socio-psychological costs for adult males, adult females and children presented in Table 10.1 shows that stigma and discrimination are broadly similar for three categories of patients. However, the same for adult female patients was marginally higher than that for adult male patients. The differential is understandable given the interpersonal interaction of each of these groups with people around them.

Table 10.1 shows that the pattern of socio-psychological experiences of defaulted patients was very much similar to those of successfully treated, though with important differences in magnitude. This assertion, however, can not be made about the two categories of patients for the phase after treatment. Whereas successfully treated patients after completing the course of treatment experienced almost the same level of social and psychological acceptance in the community as before the disease, the defaulted patients did not show this phenomenon. The defaulted TB patients during illness phase, like the successfully treated ones, faced stigma in terms of 'discrimination in food' (20.2%), 'no mixing with children' (20%).

Table 10.1: Successfully treated and defaulted TB patients (total, adult male, adult female and child) by nature of social costs due to illness by stage of Illness (before, during and after)*

Nature of social costs due to illness	*Patient type by stage of illness (%)*					
	Successfully treated			*Defaulted*		
	Stage of treatment			*Stage of treatment*		
	Before	*During*	*After*	*Before*	*During*	*After*
Total						
Discrimination within community/caste						
General	0.4	8.6	0.4	0.8	13.2	6.4
Social function/marriage	0.5	9.3	0.6	0.0	13.4	7.2
Stigma about marriage	0.8	11.0	0.8	0.8	1.8	0.0
Discrimination within family						
Discrimination in food	0.7	21.2	0.8	0.0	20.2	8.8
Separate room for living	0.9	5.5	0.8	0.8	6.4	4.8
No mixing with children	3.0	21.0	3.0	3.2	20.0	11.2
Discord in marital status	3.3	22.2	3.5	0.8	13.6	6.4
Isolated in family	0.6	2.7	0.6	0.8	4.0	4.0
Others						
Sunned by co-workers	0.6	4.0	0.8	0.8	3.2	0.8
Mental depression of the patient	0.3	18.0	0.5	0.8	14.4	4.0
Adult Male						
Discrimination within community/caste						
General	0.4	8.0	0.4	0.3	11.8	0.7
Social function/marriage	0.5	8.9	0.7	1.0	12.8	7.2
Stigma about marriage	0.7	10.8	0.7	1.0	3.9	2.0
Discrimination within family						
Discrimination in food	1.0	19.3	1.1	1.3	23.6	9.5
Separate room for living	3.1	5.9	3.3	2.0	6.2	6.2
No mixing with children	3.5	21.1	3.7	2.6	21.6	10.5
Discord in marital status	0.6	20.4	1.1	0.3	14.8	6.9
Isolated in family	0.7	10.8	0.8	0.7	7.5	4.6
Others						
Sunned by co-workers	0.5	9.4	0.8	0.0	11.8	4.6
Mental depression of the patient	1.5	18.3	0.8	0.3	16.1	7.2

Contd...

Table 10.1: Successfully treated and defaulted TB patients (total, adult male, adult female and child) by nature of social costs due to illness by stage of Illness (before, during and after)* (*Contd...*)

Nature of social costs due to illness	*Patient type by stage of illness (%)*					
	Successfully treated			*Defaulted*		
	Stage of treatment			*Stage of treatment*		
	Before	*During*	*After*	*Before*	*During*	*After*
Adult Female						
Discrimination within community/caste						
General	0.4	9.6	0.4	0.8	15.2	6.4
Social function/marriage	0.5	10.3	0.6	0.0	14.4	7.2
Stigma about marriage	0.6	3.7	0.6	0.8	0.8	0.0
Discrimination within family						
Discrimination in food	0.9	23.0	0.8	0.0	19.2	8.8
Separate room for living	3.0	5.5	3.0	0.8	6.4	4.8
No mixing with children	3.3	22.2	3.5	3.2	20.0	11.2
Discord in marital status	0.8	24.8	0.8	0.8	13.6	6.4
Isolated in family	0.6	11.1	0.8	0.8	4.0	4.0
Others						
Sunned by co-workers	0.3	6.0	0.5	0.8	3.2	0.8
Mental depression of the patient	1.3	19.6	0.9	0.8	14.4	4.0
Child						
Discrimination within community/caste						
General	0.0	4.8	0.0	0.0	13.3	13.3
Social function/marriage	0.0	5.6	0.0	0.0	13.3	13.3
Stigma about marriage	Na	Na	Na	Na	Na	Na
Discrimination within family						
Discrimination in food	0.4	13.9	0.8	6.7	26.7	20.0
Separate room for living	3.2	4.8	3.6	6.7	20.0	20.0
No mixing with children	2.8	14.3	2.4	0.0	20.0	13.3
Discord in marital status	Na	Na	Na	Na	Na	Na
Isolated in family	0	2.4	0.0	0.0	6.7	6.7
Others						
Sunned by co-workers	0	2.0	0.4	0.0	0.0	0.0
Mental depression of the patient	0.8	13.5	0.0	0.0	6.7	0.0

*Multiple responses
Na = Not applicable

'Mental depression', 'discord in marital status', 'discrimination in general and at social functions including marriages were of the same order at about 13–14%. The discrimination continued after the default on treatment, although at somewhat lower level than that during illness or treatment phase. Continued substantial discrimination in the case of defaulted patients after default on treatment might imply the presence of awareness in the people about the infective nature of the disease and associated health hazards. About 11% of defaulted patients were not able to mix with children after default on treatment. The comparative percentages for discord in marital status and discrimination in general and that in marriages at about 6–7% showed people's non-acceptance of the patients among social fold after they discontinued on medication. These facts need to be stressed frequently during the course of treatment to reduce the incidence of default among the TB patients.

More adult females than males faced general social discrimination and discrimination in marriage functions, etc. though it was not substantial but showed that females faced social wrath to a greater extent than males. By contrast, more adult males than females faced 'discrimination in food' 'no mixing with children' sunned by co-workers and 'mental depression'. The highest difference was noted in discrimination by co-workers where about 12% of defaulted adult males were sunned as compared to only about 3% of adult females. This is the reflection of the fact that more adult males were spending time out-side among co-workers than adult females who were mostly homebound. Children were also exposed to substantial social discrimination as well at family levels. In such cases after default on treatment return to earlier status was least. The pattern of discrimination against children during treatment phase was very much similar to that after the default and at the more or less same level.

10.2.2 Suspected Patients

During illness quite a few suspected TB patients faced problems such as "mental depression", "no mixing with children", "discrimination in food and residence". As illustrated by data in Table 10.2 substantially lower response rate conforming to these discriminations compared to that for successfully treated

Table 10.2: Suspected TB patients (adult male, adult female, child) by nature of social costs due to disease before and during illness*

Nature of social cost due to illness	*Patient category and stage of illness (%)*					
	Adult male		*Adult female*		*Child*	
	Before	*During*	*Before*	*During*	*Before*	*During*
Discrimination within community/caste						
General	0	3.6	0.6	0.6	0	0
Social function/marriage	0	3.6	0	0	0	0
Stigma about marriages	0	1.6	0.6	0.6	0	0
Discrimination within family	0.4	6.0	0.6	3.5	0	0
Discrimination in food	0.8	6.5	1.2	2.4	2.3	2.3
Separate room for living	0.4	4.8	1.8	3.5	2.3	2.3
No mixing with children	2.0	7.3	4.1	6.4	9.3	9.3
Discord in marital status	0	2.0	0	1.2	0	0
Isolated in family	0	3.2	0.6	2.3	0	2.3
Others						
Sunned by co-workers	0	2.4	0.6	1.2	0	0
Mental depression of the patient	0	16.1	0	9.4	0	0

*Multiple response

and defaulted patients can be explained by the status of the disease. In the former case the disease status is not confirmed therefore people around are not aware of the condition whereas in the latter two cases the disease status was confirmed. This existence of discrimination, though more of precautionary nature on the part of people around the suspected patients, might be considered a good sign that people were aware of the possible adverse consequences of catching the disease and therefore they tried to avoid people who were having symptoms of tuberculosis. The incidence of 'mental depression' in about 16% of adult males and about 9% of adult females (the highest levels noted in the survey) showed that the disease initially depressed the suspected victims. This also pointed to the fact that when patients were finally brought under the treatment it was important that counseling was done to boost their self-confidence and thus create enabling environment for quicker recovery and successful completion of the treatment course.

10.3 AWARENESS ABOUT THE DISEASE STATUS OF AND ATTITUDE TOWARD THE PATIENT

Individuals as well as families inflicted with tuberculosis prefer to conceal the disease status from others mainly to escape discrimination. In such a situation it was important to assess as to who knew about the disease condition of the patient and what was the attitude of the people who knew about it toward the patient. While the information on the first part of the question will help us to determine the degree of secrecy people would like to attach to the disease, the second part is expected to help us in quantifying the extent of people's cooperation towards patient's recovery and psychological assistance in healing and sticking to the medication regime and successfully complete the course. In this regard the survey considered five categories of people whose awareness about disease of and attitude toward patient could be useful in developing counseling programmes for TB control. These categories are: spouse, family members, relatives, friends and local people. The attitude toward patient is classified into three groups: sympathetic (SYM), discriminatory (DIS), and indifferent (IND). The findings of the survey for the total as well as for adult male, adult female and child patients are presented in Table 10.3. As explained earlier, the findings relating to successfully treated and defaulted patients are presented in Section 10.3.1 whereas those relating to the suspected patients are given in Section 10.3.2.

10.3.1 Successfully Treated and Defaulted Patients

The state of awareness about the disease status of successfully treated as well as defaulted patients as presented in Table 10.3 appears to have similar pattern. Family members and spouses knew about the disease respectively in about 94–95% and 90% of the patients. The higher incidence of the knowledge of the disease among family members compared to spouse is indicative of the fact that there were children where presence of spouse was not applicable. Further, it is clear from our data that people try to hide the disease status largely from outsiders. The incidence of awareness of the disease with reference to other three categories of people considered here is substantially lower than that observed in the case of family members and spouse. The disease status of patients was known to relatives of the successfully treated patients in about 35% of the cases. By comparison only 29% of defaulted patients confirmed that relatives were aware of their disease. Friends of only about 27% of the successfully treated as well as defaulted patients knew about the disease. Local people appear to be the last category to know about the disease status. It appears that patients and their family members and or spouses try to keep the disease status secret from local people who are in immediate neighborhood. This reflects the extent of fear that the stigma attached to disease has on the mind of people. Thus, we see that disease status was well known to spouse and family members in general (90–95% of the cases). As for others, with one exception in the case of relatives, knowing about the disease status of successfully treated patients to the extent of 35%, people in remaining categories scored less than 30% and more than 22%.

A sympathetic attitude is known to improve the immune system of the body and thus accelerate the healing process. In the case of tuberculosis this becomes more important as the treatment duration is long and the patient undergoes a lot of emotional turmoil. Our enquiry revealed that with the exception of spouse in the case of married patients very few of the patients experienced sympathetic attitude from people around them. About 84% of the successfully treated patients (86% in the case of defaulted ones) experienced sympathetic attitude of their spouses. The percentage varied from 24 to 13 in the case of family members to local people. People belonging to other categories were largely indifferent to the TB patients. Such a resigned behavior of people strengthens the case for hiding the disease status from them and increases the danger of propogation of the disease. It is surprising that even after having knowledge about the disease status the family members were not very sympathetic to the patients. The most damaging type of treatment which can be meted to a patient with detrimental result is the attitude of indifference to them.

Such an attitude is generally more destructive than the positive effect of treating them well. Since very few instances of discrimination against the patients were recorded (the maximum extent was noted in the case of successfully treated patients where local people discriminated to the extent of about 3%), the indifferent attitude was mostly the complementary part of treating them well.

The data on distribution of successfully treated and defaulted patients in the three categories (adult male, adult female, and child) presented in Table 10.3 point out some understandable differences. It may be noted that the broad pattern of awareness about disease status of patients to various categories of relatives and people is similar for adult males, adult females and children among successfully treated and defaulted patients with the exception that there is no spouse in the case of children. Also, in the case of children, because of their limited mobility out-side the household or family surroundings, relatively lower proportion among friends and local people knew about their disease status.

Knowledge of the disease status to others in the case of adult males was more frequent than in the case of adult females or children. This is the reflection of the fact that adult male patients had greater mobility than those in other categories. For example, about 38% of successfully treated adult males and about 45% of defaulted adult males confirmed that relatives were aware of their disease status. By contrast, only about 27–29% of successfully treated adult females and similar percentage of defaulted adult females confirmed that relatives and/or friends were aware of their disease status. This awareness in the case of children in both the categories of patients was still lower. The pattern of attitude toward patients in three categories of defaulted patients was more or less similar for relatives, friends and local people. The main difference in this may be noted in the case of attitude of family members where 67% had sympathetic attitude toward the sick children as opposed to 26% and 23% of sick adult males and adult females.

Table 10.3: Successfully treated and defaulted TB patients by type of relationship to those who were aware of disease status and their attitude SYM (sympathetic), DIS (discriminatory) and IND (indifferent) toward the patient*

Type of relationship to patient	Patient's category by awareness and attitude (%)									
	Successfully treated					Defaulted				
		Attitude					Attitude			
	Aware	SYM	DIS	IND	Total	Aware	SYM	DIS	IND	Total
Total										
Spouse	90.0	84.0	0.7	15.3	100.0	89.6	86.4	0.8	12.8	100.0
Family	95.0	24.0	0.3	75.7	100.0	94.4	23.2	0.0	76.8	100.0
Relatives	35.0	17.5	2.0	80.5	100.0	28.8	17.6	0.8	81.6	100.0
Friends	26.5	14.0	3.0	83.0	100.0	27.2	14.4	2.4	83.2	100.0
Local people	21.0	13.0	3.2	83.8	100.0	24.0	13.6	2.4	84.0	100.0
Adult male										
Spouse	90.2	82.5	0.6	16.9	100.0	91.1	85.2	2.6	12.2	100.0
Family	96.1	25.1	0.6	74.3	100.0	94.8	25.6	2.2	72.2	100.0
Relatives	37.7	17.2	2.9	79.9	100.0	44.9	20.7	4.6	74.7	100.0
Friends	26.0	13.0	4.3	82.7	100.0	39.7	16.1	5.9	78.0	100.0
Local people	20.5	12.7	4.0	83.3	100.0	33.1	14.8	5.9	79.3	100.0
Adult female										
Spouse	89.6	86.4	0.8	12.8	100.0	89.6	86.4	0.8	12.8	100.0
Family	94.4	23.2	0.0	76.8	100.0	94.4	23.2	0.0	76.8	100.0
Relatives	28.8	17.6	0.8	81.6	100.0	28.8	17.6	0.8	81.6	100.0
Friends	27.2	14.4	2.4	83.2	100.0	27.2	14.4	2.4	83.2	100.0
Local people	24.0	13.6	2.4	84.0	100.0	24.0	13.6	2.4	84.0	100.0
Child										
Family	98.4	16.6	0.8	82.6	100.0	80.0	66.7	0.0	33.3	100.0
Relatives	30.2	14.3	1.6	84.1	100.0	26.7	20.0	0.0	80.0	100.0
Friends	16.7	11.5	3.2	85.3	100.0	13.3	6.7	0.0	93.3	100.0
Local people	12.7	10.3	3.6	86.1	100.0	20.0	13.3	0.0	86.7	100.0

*Multiple responses

10.3.2 Suspected Patients

Like successfully treated and defaulted patients, family members and spouses were generally aware of the disease status of the patients who were suspected of TB but were not yet confirmed for the disease. About 84% of spouses and 94% of the family members were aware of the disease condition. About 31% of relatives, 20% of friends and 18% of local persons also knew about the disease condition of the patient. Spouses generally had a sympathetic attitude toward the patients (82%) but only 29% of family members showed the same temperament. The rest were indifferent. As to others, they were generally indifferent (Table 10.4).

Table 10.4: Suspected TB patients by type of relationship to those who were aware of disease status and by their attitude SYM (sympathetic), DIS (discriminatory) and IND (indifferent) toward the patient*

Type of relationship to patient	*Aware (%)*	*Attitude (%)*			
		SYM	*DIS*	*IND*	*Total*
Spouse	84.3	82.3	1.6	16.1	100.0
Family members	93.5	29.4	1.6	69.0	100.0
Relatives	30.6	18.6	2.0	79.4	100.0
Friends	20.2	11.2	2.4	86.4	100.0
Local people	17.7	9.7	1.6	88.7	100.0

*Multiple response

10.4 IMPACT ON CHILD'S EDUCATION AND REARING

10.4.1 Successfully Treated and Defaulted Patients

Tuberculosis, in the case of both the successfully treated and defaulted patients, caused an adverse impact on the education of children. This impact appeared to be somewhat more in the case of former category of patients than in the latter. Whereas in the case of former group about 25% of the patients responded that the education of children could not proceed smoothly only about 12% of defaulted patients responded in the same way. In about one percent of the cases, children were compelled to leave school and take-up employment to supplement family income. In the case of women patients, about 9% failed to carry out normal household work including taking care of children (Table 10.5).

Table 10.5 also presents our observations on impact of TB on child's education and care for three categories of patients, adult male, adult female and child. As expected, in the case of children their education got affected adversely in quite a large share of the patients (46%). TB, among adult female patients compared to male patients, appeared to cause numerically much adverse impact on child-education and care. In the case of 36% of adult female patients, education of children got adversely affected whereas in the case of 18% of such patients child-care and normal household work were adversely affected. By contrast, the disease among adult males adversely affected education of children only in 17% of the cases.

The pattern of impact of the disease in the case of defaulted patients on the education and care of children followed a similar course as that for successfully treated ones. However, the numerical magnitude of the impact was lower in the case of defaulted patients. In the case of defaulted patients about 12% reported that the education of their children was adversely affected because of the disease compared to twice as many for the successfully treated ones (25%). The comparative percentages for 'inability to take care of children and perform normal household work (in case of woman patient)' were 9 and 5. Numerically the adverse impact of the disease on the education of children and child-care as well as on normal household work in the case of defaulted patients was about one-half of that for successfully treated patients. Whether this difference in the impact has been caused by the fact that the former group spent shorter time in taking treatment than the latter one may be a subject of further study (Table 10.5).

The results of a parallel analysis of the impact of the disease on the education and care of children for defaulted adult male, adult female and child, on the line for successfully treated patients are given in Table 10.5. Here again, the pattern of impact is similar to that for the successfully treated patients with lower percentages reporting the impact. Children-education got affected adversely in 20% of the cases compared to 46% for the other group. In the case of female patients being mothers, the education of children got affected adversely in 22% of the defaulted cases compared to 35% for the other group. Further, about 16% of defaulted female patients could not take care of children and/or perform normal household work. This was not much different from the percentage for the adult females among successfully treated patients (18%) who could not perform normal household work because of the disease.

Table 10.5: Successfully treated and defaulted TB patient (adult male, adult female, child and total) by type of impact of illness on children's education and rearing*

Type of impact on child's education and rearing	*Category of patients (%)*							
	Successfully treated				*Defaulted*			
	Adult				*Adult*			
	Male	*Female*	*Child*	*Total*	*Male*	*Female*	*Child*	*Total*
Education of the children adversely affected	16.5	35.6	46.0	25.4	7.9	21.6	20.0	11.8
Inability in taking care of children and performing normal households work (incase of woman patient)	0.8	18.4	3.6	9.1	0.7	16.0	0.0	5.1
Children compelled to leave school and forced to take up employment	0.6	1.2	0.0	0.9	1.3	1.6	0.0	1.4

*Multiple responses

10.4.2 Suspected Patients

About one-fourth of the suspected TB patients in each category reported decline in their efficiency. The adverse impact of the disease on the education of children was reported mainly by children (7%) and adult female patients (4%). Impact on "not taking care of children" and "inability in performing normal household work", as expected, were reported mainly by women patients (Table 10.6). The impact of the disease in this case was

Table 10.6: Suspected TB patients (adult male, adult female and child) by type of impact of disease*

Type of impact of disease	*Percent*		
	Male	*Female*	*Child*
Decline in efficiency	25.0	25.1	27.9
Education of the children adversely affected	1.6	4.1	7.0
Inability in taking care of children and performing normal household work	2.0	35.7	0.0

*Multiple response

numerically quite low compared to that for successfully treated or defaulted ones probably because of the uncertainty of the status and smaller period of exposure to the disease.

11

Service: Quality and Satisfaction

11.1 SCOPE AND CONTENTS

The success of tuberculosis control programme, like any other people oriented one, largely depends upon the productive blend of service providers on the one hand and the service users on the other. Chapters 7 through 10 of this book have covered the characteristics of service users of RNTCP. The present chapter summarizes the findings in respect of selected parameters of service providers active in the control and treatment of TB. The quality of these services as assessed from the provider's perspective needed some validation from the point of view of service users. Hence, the study on the quality of services available considered a sample of TB patients currently under treatment at selected DOTS and other centers. The profile of, along with the perception of quality of service by, the patients receiving treatment from the service providers selected and interviewed in the sample are also summarized in this chapter.

For this purpose our sample considered 100 service providers. The in-charge of each of these units was interviewed to collect data regarding selected characteristics of human resource and available facilities for providing services to the patients. The survey covered four factors which could help/harm the patronization of services by patients assuming they had a choice. These were:

- Distance from the nearest bus stand
- Status of surroundings
- Type of facilities available
- Category and behavior of human resource at the center

To cover the current patients, an exit interview of each of 2,500 patients specifically selected as explained in methodology (Chapter 7) and visiting the 100 service providers was carried out. In the case of service users, the exit interview covered the following aspects

- Patient's profile covering gender, marital status, literacy and employment status
- Awareness and choice about DOTS center
- Other hospitals visited earlier
- Progress status
- Distance of DOTS center
- Waiting place
- Waiting time
- Behavior of staff
- Facilities at the service provider
- Quality of service given by service provider.

11.2 SERVICE PROVIDERS

11.2.1 Category of Service Providers

Table 11.1 provides the distribution of service providers by category and type. Of the 100 service providers considered for this study, 76 were DOTS centers exclusively run for the purpose of treatment of TB, 9 were DOTS centers run with the assistance of NGOs. Further, 8 service providers were from government hospitals and remaining 7 were attached to private hospitals/dispensaries.

Thus, of the 100 service providers surveyed, 76 were exclusively for treatment of TB. The remaining ones were working as part of hospitals or other health facilities.

Table 11.1: Service providers by category and type

Category	*Percent*
DOTS centers	38
Dispensary having DOTS center	38
DOTS centers run with NGO assistance	9
Govt. hospitals	8
Private hospital/dispensaries	7
Type	
Yes only for TB	76
Combined with other health facilities	24
Total	100

11.2.2 Distance

Distance from the nearest public sector transport system is critical for the success of a programme such as tuberculosis control. Shorter distance from the bus stand will be quite useful in facilitating the visit by patients to these centers on a daily basis in general and at least in the beginning of the medication in particular. In this respect it may be noted that the government has a policy to locate these service centers at convenient places. Table 11.2 provides the details about the distance of the service provider from the nearest bus stop. It may be noted that about 21% of service providers were just adjacent to a nearby bus stand and an additional about 58% of them were located within about one km. of a nearby bus stand. Thus, about 80% of the

Table 11.2: Distance of service providers from nearest bus stand

Distance (nearest km)	*Percent*	
0	21	
1	58	
2	15	
> 2	6	
Total	100	
	Yes	**No**
Whether easy to walk from the bus stand (%)	63	27

facilities were located within comfortable walking distance from the nearest bus stand. More than 20% of the service providers were located at a distance of 2 kilometers or more from the nearest bus stand. Although almost 80% of the service providers were located within one kilometer of the nearest bus stand, only 63% of them were considered "easy to walk" from the nearest bus stand. Opening of more DOTS centers and locating these strategically would be necessary to ameliorate the difficulties faced by patients, who were generally poor in health and financial resources, in accessing these centers.

11.2.3 Surroundings

Next to the distance to be covered from the nearest bus stand, it is the surroundings of the center for service provider which may count in quality service. Table 11.3 presents the results on the status of cleanliness of the surroundings of premises housing various DOTS centers as well as other service providers included in the study. Status of cleanliness has been reported as a matter of concern by the service providers. Only one in five service providers could consider the surrounding as clean. By contrast, about three-tenths of them considered the status of cleanliness around the premises as dirty or very dirty. Only about one-half of the providers surveyed thought the cleanliness around the center was tolerable. Our visit to some of the selected centers revealed the poor state of cleanliness. It would be desirable for project management to look into this and implement measures for improvement of the existing status.

Table 11.3: Surroundings of the service provider by state of cleanliness

State of Cleanliness	*Percent*
Very clean	1
Clean	20
Tolerable	51
Dirty	23
Very dirty	5
Total	100

11.2.4 Facilities

The third important factor that needs consideration for a good set-up is the physical facilities, namely, waiting place and utilities, etc. available for use by patients. The details on facilities available on the premises of the service providers as gathered from them are presented in Table 11.4. It may be noted that about 84% of the service providers had some covered waiting area for the patients. This comprised of pucca room (38%), verandah (28%) and tin/thatch shade (18%). In about 16% of the cases patients were required to wait in the open. Separate dispensing room and consulting room were available with 86% and 70% of the service providers respectively.

Facility for drinking water was available with about three-fourths of the service providers (74%). It was a matter of concern for one-quarter of the service providers that patients had to make provision themselves for drinking water in order to take the medicines on the spot. Similar was the situation with toilet facility. About 72% of service providers had provision for toilets for males whereas 5 percentage points fewer of them had toilets for females. To provide a quality service, it would be imperative for the programme managers to provide toilet and drinking water facilities at each center.

Table 11.4: Facilities available with service providers

Facilities	*Percent*	
Waiting facility		
Pucca room	38	
Verandah	28	
Tin/thatch	18	
Open Space	16	
Total	**100**	
Other facilities	**Yes**	**No**
Consulting room	69	31
Dispensing room	86	14
Drinking water	74	26
Toilet Male	72	28
Toilet Female	67	33

11.2.5 Human Resource

The distribution of available human resource in post at the time of survey who could provide services to patients by number and category is presented in Table 11.5.

Table 11.5: Service provider by number and category of human resource available

	Category of human resource (%)			
Number of staff	*Doctor*	*Nurse*	*Technician*	*Helper*
0	35	52	36	87
1	28	34	48	7
2 or more	37	14	16	6
Total	**100**	**100**	**100**	**100**

It may be noted that only 65% of service providers had at least one doctor in post at the time of survey. It was surprising to note that almost one-third of the service centers were functioning without a doctor to take care of patients. A similar situation was noted for technicians (64% in post). The situation with nursing staff was even worse. Nurses were in position only in 48% of the service centers. Only 13% of service providers had a helper. This shows a severe shortage of human resource to service the patients at DOTS centers.

11.3 EXIT INTERVIEWS

In order to validate the claims made by service providers it was necessary to assess the views of the current patients regarding the quality of service provided by them. The findings from the exit interviews of 2,500 current TB patients are discussed in the following sections. We have also included the profile of current patients to assess the socio-economic background of those patients who visit the DOTS and other centers catering to such patients.

11.3.1 Gender

Table 11.6 gives the distribution by gender of current TB patients contacted through exit interview. About 54% of patients visiting these centers and interviewed were males and remaining 46% were females. It may be recalled that the percentage of males and females among those who successfully completed treatment was 53 and 47 respectively. The closeness of the gender composition of patients in the two categories shows some sort of stability in the prevalence of TB among males and females who visit the DOTS centers.

Table 11.6: Current TB patients by gender

Gender	*Percent*
Male	54
Female	46
Total	**100**

11.3.2 Marital Status

Table 11.7 presents the distribution of current TB patients according to marital status. Of all the current TB patients attending DOTS centers, about 39% were unmarried. Married ones comprised about 60% of the total. Widower and separated formed a negligible share with less than 0.6%.

Table 11.7: Distribution of current TB patients by marital status

Marital status	*Percent*
Unmarried	39.0
Married	60.4
Widow/widower	0.3
Separated	0.3
Total	**100.0**

11.3.3 Literacy

Table 11.8, the distribution of current TB patients according to literacy status, shows that of the current patients about 15% were illiterate and 6% could just read and write. The majority of them (63%) had education between primary to matriculation levels. Only about 2% had education up to graduation level.

Table11.8: Distribution of current TB patients by literacy/education level

Literacy/education level	*Percent*
Illiterate	15.4
Read and write	6.0
Primary	29.0
Middle	34.4
Matriculation	13.2
Graduate	2.0
Total	**100.0**

11.3.4 Working Status

The distribution of current TB patients by working status is presented in Table 11.9. About 37% were working and rest 63% were not working. Share of working patients comprised of 18% on daily wages and somewhat higher percentage (19%) on monthly salary. Of those not working, majority were housewives and students. The composition of current patients by working/ not-working status is very similar to that of the successfully treated ones but very different from that of defaulted ones. By implication it may point to the fact that the current patients were very likely to successfully complete the treatment course.

Table 11.9: Current TB patients by working status

Working status	*Percentage*
Working on daily wages	18.1
Working on monthly wages	18.8
Not working	63.1
Total	**100.0**

11.3.5 Awareness about and choice of DOTS Center

The distribution of current patients according to who advised them to choose the DOTS center for treatment presented in Table 11.10 showed the importance of the role played by the family in the selection of the center. It may be noted that as high as 80% of patients chose to avail the services from DOTS centers as per advice of family members whereas only 12% of them did that on their own. Advice of relatives, friends as well as that of medical professionals also helped them in choosing a DOTS center. The respective percentages may be noted as 31, 31 and 12. The significantly high percentage of patients getting advice from family members to attend the DOTS center shows that family can play a very important role in tuberculosis control. It may be pointed that the large percentage of patients are adult females and children where family can definitely play the decisive role in the RNTCP.

Table 11.10: Current patient's choice of DOTS center being attended by source of advice*

Choice helped by	*Percent*
Own knowledge	11.6
Advice of family members	79.2
Advice of friends	31.0
Advice of relatives	30.7
Advice of medical professional	12.0

*Multiple response

11.3.6 Other Hospitals Visited

To understand the treatment seeking behavior of current TB patients it is useful to know whether they visited other hospitals for treatment before coming to the present service provider. Table 11.11 shows that about one-fourth of current patients did in fact visit other hospitals for treatment before coming to present DOTS centers.

Table 11.11: Current TB patients by status of earlier visit to any other service provider for the present disease

Status of earlier visit to any other service provider	*Percent*
Yes	24.7
No	75.3
Total	**100.0**

11.3.7 Progress Status

The results on progress with the treatment as perceived by the current patients are presented in Table 11.12. It is encouraging to note that as high as 97% of current patients reported that the progress was satisfactory.

Table 11.12: Current TB patients by perceived status of progress made during treatment

Perceived progress made during treatment	*Percent*
Too short to comment	3.1
Satisfactory	96.8
Not satisfactory	0.1
Total	**100.0**

11.3.8 Distance of DOTS Center

Location of DOTS centers in relation to the residence of users plays an important role in facilitating the compliance of patients. There are two aspects in this respect. One, it relates to the location of the center from the nearest bus stand and two, the location of the center in relation to the residence of users. The first aspect we analyzed in the previous section while looking at the responses from the service providers. The second aspect we will investigate in this section. Table 11.13 gives the results on the distance of service centers from the residence of the patients. The distance of the service centers from the residences of the current patients was within 1 km for 54%, 1–2 km for 34% and more than 2 km for 12% of the respondents. If we consider that the location of the center at a distance of less than two kilometers is a convenient one for use by patients, (this distance may be covered by a public transport system as well), we find that as much as close to 90% of the centers were located within two kilometers from the residence of the users. These findings are quite consistent with those recorded in the case of successfully treated and defaulted patients (*see* Table 8.7) where 8–9% were located at more than two kilometers from the nearest DOTS center.

Table 11.13: Current TB patients by distance of DOTS center from their residence

Distance of DOTS center from patient's residence	*Percent*
1 km	54.1
2 km	34.3
>2 km	11.6
Total	**100.0**

11.3.9 Waiting Place

After reaching the center, there are two aspects which need consideration. One relates to the waiting place and other to waiting time spent in getting the services delivered. This aspects is investigated in this and the following section. The results on type of waiting place for patients available with the service providers are given in Table 11.14. The waiting place in the form of a room was available for only about 38% of the respondents. About 45% of the current patients had to wait in a Verandah whereas about 16% of them had to wait only in the open. The use of open space and verandah for waiting place, particularly in Delhi summer, by patients who are already weak could be quite taxing. Since as much as 62% of the patients had to wait for services in this type of place, it might be useful to consider some mitigating measures.

Table 11.14: Current TB patients by type of waiting space available at the service provider

Type of waiting place available at the service provider	Percent
Open space*	16.8
Waiting room	38.4
Verandah	44.8
Total	**100.0**

*This includes those with tin shed.

11.3.10 Waiting Time

The results on waiting time spent are given in Table 11.15. Large number of patients (about 90%) could wait less than or equal to 15 minutes for collection of medicines. Only a small share (about 10%) had to wait longer than 15 minutes for the same purpose. By contrast, about two-thirds of current patients had to wait for consultation for less than or equal to 15 minutes. The remaining ones had to wait longer than that. Consultation and collection of medicines, on the average, appear to take about one-half hour for every patient.

Table 11.15: Current TB patients by waiting time and type of service utilized

Waiting time (min)	Type of service utilized (%)	
	Consultation	Medicines collection
<10	3.1	5.0
10	25.9	57.6
15	34.7	27.8
20	13.9	3.5
30	14.4	2.6
>30	8.0	3.5
Total	100.0	100.0
Average (min)	18	14

11.3.11 Behavior of Staff

Sympathetic behavior of staff at the center is expected to yield satisfied and happy users. Such an act might also help patients to be more conscious of their condition and turn them into proactive users. These interactions are expected to improve the success of tuberculosis control programme. It was in this light that the survey attempted to assess the perception of patients about the behavior of staff at the DOTS centers they were attending. We considered the staff in three categories. These were: doctor, paramedical staff and health educator. Data presented in Table 11.16 show that a sympathetic behavior of doctor and health educator was reported respectively by 84%

Table 11.16: Current TB patients by perceived behavior of staff by category

Perceived Behavior	Category of staff (%)		
	Doctor	Paramedical	Health educator
Very Sympathetic	2.5	1.6	16.1
Sympathetic	84.1	30.8	78.1
Indifferent	0.6	1.2	3.9
Not caring	0.0	64.5	1.9
NR	12.8	1.9	0.0
Total	**100.0**	**100.0**	**100.0**

and 78% of the current patients. By contrast, the sympathetic behavior by paramedical staff was reported by only 31% of the current TB patients. The incidence of very sympathetic behavior shown by doctor or paramedical staff was almost negligible. By contrast, close to 16% of the current patients found the behavior of health educator as "very sympathetic". Somewhat two-thirds of the current patients felt that paramedical staff's behavior was that of "not caring" type. To improve compliance by patients and thereby increase in efficiency in RNTCP it may be useful to consider "motivational training" for the paramedical staff.

11.3.12 Facilities at the Service Provider

The availability of waiting room at the service providers was reported by 63% of current patients. This response was in agreement with that given by service providers where it was indicated that 66% of them had a provision for waiting place in the form of a room or a verandah (Table 11.4). The availability of tin/thatched shade, reported by 18% of the service providers, was not considered good enough by the current patients. To increase patient's satisfaction regarding the waiting place it may be necessary to augment the physical facilities of DOTS centers in all respects including those for waiting, sanitary and hygiene ones. About 82% respondents confirmed the availability of drinking water whereas 78% of them reported that toilets were available. These figures are somewhat similar to those reported by the service providers. Nearly all the current patients found the "waiting time" reasonable and comfortable (Table 11.17).

Table 11.17: Current TB patients by type of facilities available for patients at service provider

Facilities available		*Percent*
Waiting room*		62.5
Toilet		77.7
Drinking water		81.9
Waiting time:	Long	0.9
	Reasonable	98.3
Waiting hours:	Tolerable	97.1
	Not tolerable	1.9

*This includes Verandah.

11.3.13 Quality of Services given by Service Providers

Most of the respondents (about 88%) found the quality of service provided by the service centers as good or better. Majority of the remainder found the service satisfactory. A negligible percentage of respondents found the service poor (Table 11.18).

Table 11.18: Current TB patients by perceived quality of services given by service provider

Perceived quality of service	*Percent*
Excellent	0.6
Very good	13.2
Good	74.6
Satisfactory	10.4
Poor	0.3

11.3.14 Behavior of Patient in respect of Taking Treatment

Regularity in taking medicines is a key element in tuberculosis control programme and it is emphasized on the patients after registration. It is heartening to find that as high as 99% of patients reported that they were regular in treatment as well as in getting medicines on time. About 88% patients were taking the medicines on the spot and rest of them were taking the medicine home. Details are given in Table 11.19.

Table 11.19: Current TB patient's behavior in respect of taking medicines

Behavior of patients in respect of taking medicine	*Percent*
Regular in treatment	99.5
Getting medicines regularly	99.4
Taking medicines on time	99.5
Taken on spot	87.5
Taken at home	12.6
Taking as advised	83.3

Index